DATE DUE			
MAR 0 9 1994			

DEMCO 38-297

CONTRAST MEDIA IN MAGNETIC RESONANCE IMAGING

CONTRAST MEDIA IN MAGNETIC RESONANCE IMAGING

A CLINICAL APPROACH

Edited by

VAL M. RUNGE, M.D.

Rosenbaum Professor of Diagnostic Radiology
Director of the Magnetic Resonance Imaging
  and Spectroscopy Center
University of Kentucky
Lexington, Kentucky

WITH 4 ADDITIONAL CONTRIBUTORS

J.B. LIPPINCOTT COMPANY
Philadelphia

New York   London   Hagerstown

Acquisitions Editor: Peg Forster
Designer: Doug Smock
Production Coordinator: P. M. Gordon Associates
Compositor: Omegatype
Printer/Binder: Halliday Lithograph Corporation

Portions of the chapters in this book are reprinted with permission from *Topics in Magnetic Resonance Imaging,* vol. 3, no. 2, March 1991.

6 5 4 3 2 1

Library of Congress Cataloging-in-Publication Data

Contrast media in magnetic resonance imaging : a clinical
  approach / edited by Val M. Runge : with 4 additional
  contributors.
      p. cm.
    Includes bibliographical references and index.
    ISBN 0–397–51270–8
    1. Magnetic resonance imaging. 2. Contrast media. I. Runge,
Val M.
    [DNLM: 1. Contrast Media. 2. Magnetic Resonance Imaging.
WN 445 C764]
RC78.7.N83C67 1991
616.07′548—dc20
DNLM/DLC
for Library of Congress   91–41008
                                                      CIP

The authors and publisher have exerted every effort to ensure that drug selection and dosage set forth in this text are in accord with current recommendations and practice at the time of publication. However, in view of ongoing research, changes in government regulations, and the constant flow of information relating to drug therapy and drug reactions, the reader is urged to check the package insert for each drug for any change in indications and dosage and for added warnings and precautions. This is particularly important when the recommended agent is a new or infrequently employed drug.

To my two daughters, Valerie and Sadie, and my wife B. J., with all
my love

CONTRIBUTORS

Graeme M. Bydder, M.D.

Professor of Diagnostic Radiology, Royal Post Graduate Medical School, Hammersmith Hospital, London, England

Bruce L. Dean, M.D.

Southwest Neuro-Imaging, Phoenix, Arizona

John E. Kirsch, Ph.D.

Assistant Professor of Diagnostic Radiology and Biomedical Engineering, Director of Research for the Magnetic Resonance Imaging and Spectroscopy Center, University of Kentucky, Lexington, Kentucky

Charles Lee, M.D.

Associate Professor of Diagnostic Radiology, University of Kentucky, Lexington, Kentucky

Val M. Runge, M.D.

Professor of Diagnostic Radiology, Director of the Magnetic Resonance Imaging and Spectroscopy Center, University of Kentucky, Lexington, Kentucky

PREFACE

Dedicated research in contrast media for magnetic resonance imaging (MRI) began in 1981 and has spanned the last ten years. Pharmaceutical development in MRI offered an opportunity not matched by x-ray-based modalities, given in particular the lower doses (grams per kilogram) required for enhancement. Although only one agent (gadopentetate dimeglumine) is currently approved by the U.S. Food and Drug Administration, clinical trials of several additional gadolinium chelates are nearing completion. This group includes gadoteridol, a nonionic agent with sufficiently low toxicity to permit high-dose applications. Despite the relative newness of the field, contrast-agent use has already begun to dominate head and spine imaging. Magnetic resonance (MR) also offers the opportunity for development of more tissue-specific contrast media. For example, both hepatobiliary and particulate agents have been designed and have recently undergone clinical trials.

The explosive growth encountered in contrast-media development and MR itself has been unparalleled in diagnostic imaging. Although development has not yet plateaued, it is now possible, because of the large clinical database available, to begin summarizing and consolidating observations with respect to applications and technique.

This textbook presents an overview of basic principles regarding MRI contrast media, a review of specific applications in the head and spine, a survey of clinical experience in the body, and a perspective of future development. The clinical material presented details the common applications of contrast media in MRI clinical practice. The use of gadopentetate dimeglumine or other similar gadolinium chelates in head MRI is now approaching the levels of use of iodinated agents in head computed tomography (CT). Application of contrast media in spine imaging is common, but less frequent than that in the head. Improved sensitivity for both intradural and extradural disease has been shown, with additional application in the evaluation of disk disease. Utilization in body imaging remains limited, although this represents the largest area for potential growth in the next few years. It is anticipated that the introduction of new pulse sequences, enabling image acquisition during suspended respiration and first pass studies, will enhance the use of intravenous contrast media in organs outside the central nervous system.

In addition to the success demonstrated in clinical application by renally excreted gadolinium chelates, numerous other MR contrast agents (both oral and intravenous) are currently under laboratory and clinical investigation. Some are nonspecific extracellular agents; others are targeted for a specific tissue or organ system. These agents, if approved for clinical use, will without doubt expand further the clinical utility of MRI. The availability of an oral contrast agent for opacification of the gastrointestinal tract, combined with the advent of fast imaging sequences, will also likely lead to the use of body MRI as the screening procedure of choice.

This textbook is intended for both physicians and basic scientists and covers the current clinical usage of contrast media. Most applications involve improved lesion detection or tissue characterization, although considerable potential exists for supplementation with biochemical and physiologic data. The clinical material presented provides the reader with an understanding of current applications, ensuring informed use of contrast media and appropriate interpretation of studies.

Acknowledgment. This text was made possible by the substantial contributions of both staff and physicians at Tufts University and the University of Kentucky. Lisa Miller, in particular, was of great help, especially with editing during the final publication process.

Val M. Runge

CONTENTS

Basic Principles of Magnetic Resonance Contrast Agents

John E. Kirsch

A contrast agent employed in an imaging procedure serves to improve diagnostic sensitivity and specificity by altering the intrinsic properties of tissues that influence the fundamental mechanisms of contrast. Strategic localization of the agent can regionally change the tissue properties, thereby resulting in preferential enhancement. In this respect, magnetic resonance imaging (MRI) is unique among all diagnostic modalities. Whereas most types of imaging depend on one inherent property, MRI contrast is influenced by numerous nuclear magnetic resonance (NMR) properties of the tissues. This has led to an area of pharmaceutical chemistry that introduces many avenues of development and new challenges in the search for optimal contrast agents in MRI.

In addition to the complexities posed to the NMR chemist, the use of contrast agents in an imaging procedure is equally multifaceted to the MRI radiologist. The interdependence of multiple NMR properties on the signal and contrast of an image can significantly differ, based on the protocol chosen by the radiologist. Furthermore, in a multitude of different applications, MRI has seen a rapid growth that has expanded its usefulness, particularly in recent years. Techniques have, in themselves, introduced new types of contrast. The use of contrast agents in MRI presents a formidable challenge to the radiologist who must understand its mechanism of enhancement, the dependence of the altered NMR property on imaging parameters, and its role in the overall contrast of a given MRI technique.

The idea of contrast enhancement in NMR has been investigated as early as the pioneering work of Bloch[1] on the NMR phenomenon. The influence of paramagnetic ions on the relaxation of protons was first theorized by Bloembergen and colleagues[2] in 1948 and, eventually, led to the first imaging experiments performed with a paramagnetic agent by Young and co-workers.[3] Contrast agents have since expanded beyond paramagnetic relaxation enhancement and, most recently, have provided the means for MRI to obtain functional information with the advent of ultrafast imaging methods.

The purpose of this discussion is to provide a better understanding of the basic principles and issues involved in the development and use of contrast agents in MRI. Because of the wealth of information and for the sake of clarity, rigorous theory will not be presented. Rather, a conceptual presentation will be given. There are numerous types of contrast agents, strategies, and applications that exist and that are beyond the scope of this chapter. Instead, the goal is to present the underlying general principles behind them so that an understanding can be attained of how and why contrast agents are used in MRI.

GENERAL REQUIREMENTS FOR MAGNETIC RESONANCE CONTRAST AGENT DESIGN

In the design and development of an MRI contrast agent, certain criteria are followed. The extension of MRI to agent-enhanced diagnostics requires that the agent be biocompatible as well as enhancing. The criteria can be categorized in a general way as for any standard pharmaceutical used in a diagnostic procedure.

CONTRAST-ENHANCING MECHANISM

In general, the pharmaceutical must possess the ability to manipulate the parameters that influence the contrast-forming mechanism. This is a primary goal in any contrast-enhanced imaging procedure. Magnetic resonance imaging is unique in this manner because the image intensity is dependent on more than one parameter. Thus, more than one strategy can be pursued in the development of an MRI agent to enhance contrast. The efficiency will depend on the ability to alter the contrast parameter, or parameters, at a given concentration. This is an important issue when addressing dose and toxicity. The agent should be efficient enough that it can significantly alter the contrast mechanism at sufficiently low concentrations. Finally, the effects of the agent on the signal and contrast should be reproducible from examination to examination.

IN VIVO TARGETING AND TISSUE SPECIFICITY

For the agent to be of diagnostic value, it should be chemically versatile so that it can be bound to other compounds as an in vivo probe to permit selective tissue localization. True targeting is rarely achieved and usually compromises other criteria in the pharmaceutical design. The diagnostic usefulness of a contrast-enhanced MR examination will depend on the concentration of the agent delivered locally to the desired tissue as well as the selectivity of the distribution relative to other tissues. Of equal importance are the temporal characteristics of the distribution. The enhancing agent must remain for a period in the targeted tissue at sufficient levels that the imaging procedure can be carried out and enhancement can be achieved, ultimately leading to increased tissue specificity.

STABILITY

The substance should possess shelf stability and be capable of easy storage, preferably in a form suitable for immediate use. More importantly, the agent should be stable in vivo. Breakdown of the substance after administration can alter its targeting characteristics and potentially lead to increased toxicity.

EXCRETABILITY AND TISSUE CLEARANCE

Although the agent must possess temporal characteristics amenable for targeting, it must also be designed to be excreted, preferably within a few hours of administration. The complete clearance of the agent from the body, either by hepatobiliary or renal pathways, is desirable for overall low toxicity. Long-term retention of the agent can potentially lead to chronic toxic effects.

TOXICITY

The agent developed to satisfy other criteria must ultimately stand up to the scrutiny of toxicity evaluation for it to be acceptable for clinical use. Acute as well as chronic toxicity is related to the in vivo stability of the agent, its biodistribution, and its tissue clearance behavior. The substance must be evaluated for mutagenicity, teratogenicity, carcinogenicity, and immunogenicity, to determine safe dose levels. In addition, the process of testing must include considerations of acute lethal toxicity (LD_{50} values), sublethal toxicities (including effects on the cardiovascular and neurologic

systems), and subacute toxicity (including chemical alterations in the blood and urine, and histologic evidence of damage in multiple organs). Finally, the agent must ultimately be such that it can be administered at low enough doses to be nontoxic without compromising its enhancement capability.

MAGNETIC RESONANCE CONTRAST MECHANISMS

Above all else, a contrast agent must be evaluated for its effectiveness in enhancing image contrast between normal and diseased tissue or yield functional information about an organ or blood flow. Therefore, the mechanisms of contrast enhancement must be understood. Magnetic resonance imaging is unique among all diagnostic-imaging modalities in this respect, which is clearly seen by first examining computed tomography (CT) and its contrast mechanisms.

In CT, an x-ray beam is attenuated through matter. A single tissue parameter, the mass absorption coefficient (μ), determines the degree of attenuation and is dependent on the elemental composition of the tissue, specifically, the electron density and its effective atomic number Z. Larger values of μ (and Z) lead to greater reduction in the beam intensity, and contrast is derived from the differences in μ between neighboring tissues. It follows then that the mechanism for contrast enhancement in CT involves simply the manipulation of μ. Introduction of a high-Z material, such as iodine, can increase μ, thereby enhancing the contrast through greater attenuation of the x-ray beams. Strategic localization of an iodinated contrast agent, therefore, will increase diagnostic specificity and tissue conspicuity.

Unlike CT, however, MRI is neither quantitative nor parametrically singular in its contrast mechanism. Image contrast in MRI is based on differences in NMR signal between tissues. What makes MRI fundamentally unique from CT and other imaging modalities is that this signal is not only multiparametric in the NMR properties of the tissues, but also multiparametric in the method of its measurement. This cannot be overstated in its importance both in conventional and contrast-enhanced MRI. Although substantial differences in their NMR properties may exist between two tissues, even in the absence of contrast agents, inappropriate selection of the method of measurement and its associated parameters can lead to substantially reduced contrast. Certainly, this same consequence can arise when contrast-enhancing agents are introduced. This discussion will be presented later in more detail.

The determinants of signal and contrast in MRI are numerous. Spin density (ρ), susceptibility (χ), relaxation (T1 and T2), and motion (diffusion and perfusion), all are characteristics of tissue that influence the

NMR signal and are, in theory, parameters that can be manipulated pharmacologically for the purposes of contrast enhancement. It will be seen that the most promising agents alter the relaxation of tissues, and the bulk of the research and development of MRI contrast media has been in this area. For understanding, however, other parameters will be briefly discussed in terms of their potential as MRI contrast enhancement mechanisms.

Spin Density

The NMR signal in imaging originates from hydrogen nuclei (protons). The maximum potential signal coming from any one given tissue is directly proportional to the fraction of protons that contribute to this signal and constitutes the parameter, *spin density*, or ρ. Most protons in human tissues are associated with water, whether it is bulk, structured, or bound. Most tissues typically consist of 60% to 80% water. Moreover, water protons far outnumber other protons in organic components. Since the water content in tissue is relatively constant, little variation exists between tissues for hydrogen content or spin density. Signal, using any method of measurement, is directly proportional to spin density, and alteration of ρ to induce contrast enhancement would require significant changes in the water content (either by selective hydration or dehydration) to be diagnostically useful, usually making this an impractical approach. Furthermore, relaxation characteristics of water are so largely different from most tissues that changes in water content will also produce substantial changes in relaxation parameters (T1 and T2). Nevertheless, ordinary water has been investigated as an aid in delineation of the alimentary tract.[4]

Nonproton agents, inducing an absence of hydrogen density in their presence, lead to signal decrease and, therefore, a signal-negating form of enhancement (negative enhancement). One such agent, perfluorohexylbromide (PFHB), has been initially investigated and showed some clinical usefulness for gastrointestinal (GI) tract imaging.[5] However, such strategies tend to be restrictive in applicability and have received limited attention.

Susceptibility

All forms of matter, whether solid, liquid, or gas, possess the macroscopic property of magnetic susceptibility (χ). This parameter describes the ability of the medium to become magnetized in the presence of an external magnetic field. Here χ is defined as the ratio of induced magnetization to that of the applied field. Substances can be grouped by χ into four main categories: diamagnetism, paramagnetism, superparamagnetism, and ferromagnetism. Generally speaking, diamagnetic substances have small, negative susceptibilities ($\chi < 0$), paramagnetics have positive susceptibilities ($\chi > 0$), and superparamagnetic and ferromagnetic materials have large positive susceptibilities ($\chi \gg 0$).

Most organic and inorganic compounds and biologic tissues are diamagnetic ($\chi < 0$). All other substances possess a diamagnetic component, but are dominated by either paramagnetic or ferromagnetic properties. The negative susceptibility of diamagnetism, although weak, induces a negative magnetization that opposes the external field, decreasing the total resultant field induced within the medium. Diamagnetism is exhibited in materials that have the great majority of their electrons paired, thereby interacting only weakly with the external field, according to Lenz's law; and diamagnetism generates little or no magnetic moment. Therefore, diamagnetic susceptibility by itself has little effect in NMR and is of little interest as a contrast-enhancing mechanism as well. It has, however, been seen to produce small decreases in T1 relaxation and is speculated to be the reason for high signal intensities seen in some body fluids on T1-weighted spin echo images.[6] It has also been proposed by one group to use diamagnetic clay minerals, not as a susceptibility agent per se, but rather, as substances introduced to absorb water molecules, thereby changing regional relaxivity.[7]

In paramagnetic substances ($\chi > 0$), the predominant magnetic effect arises from unpaired electron spins that generate individual atomic or molecular magnetic moments. These moments are independent of each other in the absence of an external field, and they are isotropic and randomly oriented. In the presence of an external field, a net directional magnetic moment is induced that tends to align parallel to the applied field. If enough unpaired electrons exist in the medium, paramagnetism will dominate over diamagnetic effects. When the external field is eliminated, the collective magnetic moment will characteristically lose the alignment, tending once again toward randomly oriented and independent moments associated with the unpaired electron spins.

Use of paramagnetic ions overwhelmingly dominates the research and development of MRI contrast agents. However, the enhancement mechanism is not usually associated directly with their magnetic susceptibility. The presence of paramagnetic ions in tissues strongly influences the relaxation properties of protons which in turn leads to changes in tissue contrast. Paramagnetics and their relaxation effects will be dealt with in a later section. A few recent studies, however, have indicated that, with appropriate selection of the MRI method of measurement and parameters, paramagnetic agents can be used for susceptibility contrast enhancement, particularly if employed at high-dose levels.[8,9]

If a large number of unpaired spins reside together in a solid phase or crystalline structure, called domains, very large values of χ are produced, since their magnetic moments will couple collectively to yield larger magnetic moments. These substances are considered superparamagnetics and ferromagnetics ($\chi \gg 0$). Existence of these domains defines the two classifications. They are distinguished, however, by whether neighboring domains interact with, or reside independently of, each other. This primarily depends on the size and nature of the solid.

Superparamagnetics are individual particles large enough to be domains but small enough to be singular, randomly oriented, and noninteracting. In an applied field, these domains align with the field, setting up a very large and positive net magnetization; in the absence of the field they lose the magnetization and return to random orientations, similar to paramagnetic substances with their smaller dipole moments.

Ferromagnetic substances, on the other hand, are collections of interacting domains in a larger crystalline form that retains their magnetization by hysteresis when an external field is applied and then removed. Superparamagnetic and ferromagnetic substances have also been widely investigated as contrast agents, particularly in recent years.[10–12] Unlike paramagnetics, however, their mechanism of contrast enhancement is more directly associated with susceptibility than with relaxation.

In a perfectly homogeneous medium possessing a uniform susceptibility distribution at the molecular level, the effect of susceptibility on the MR signal is negligible. If, however, two regions of tissue exist with sufficiently different χ values, the MR signal will be influenced by susceptibility in the form of a signal loss at the interface. This occurs because both tissues experience different magnetic fields owing to their different susceptibilities, resulting in a small magnetic field gradient that becomes induced at the interface. Transverse spins in this region will experience slightly different precessional frequencies and potentially will become dephased, producing a net magnetization loss and subsequent decrease in the signal at the interface. In the absence of any externally introduced agent, susceptibility poses little influence on either signal or contrast, since most tissues possess similar χ values, except at boundaries of large susceptibility differences, such as air–tissue interfaces. However, in some circumstances, susceptibility-induced contrast has been seen owing to the presence of ferritin in hemochromatosis, for example, and in deoxyhemoglobin, methemoglobin, and hemosiderin in hemorrhage.[13,14]

When a superparamagnetic or ferromagnetic substance, such as iron oxide, is introduced into tissues, highly localized susceptibility changes occur. Each domain (superparamagnetic contrast agent) or collection of domains (ferromagnetic contrast agent) possesses a microscopic region of large-field inhomogeneity owing

to their high susceptibility relative to the surrounding tissue. This induces a spin dephasing and subsequent signal loss similar to what occurs at tissue–air interfaces, except that the susceptibility mechanism occurs at a much smaller scale, typically within the dimensions of an imaging voxel. Consequently, localized image intensity losses occur in the regions containing the negatively enhancing agent. Spin dephasing is caused by a number of mechanisms. T2 relaxation is a spin-dephasing process, resulting from the molecular environment, and will be presented in the following section. The total dephasing time, known as T2*, is a combination of T2 effects and other dephasing processes of which susceptibility is a major contributing factor. Usually, image contrast related to susceptibility, particularly when a contrast agent is used to enhance susceptibility, is referred to as T2* contrast.

Use of susceptibility as a contrast or contrast-enhancing mechanism is greatly dependent on the method of measurement. Accentuation or suppression of susceptibility effects is possible by varying the type of MRI protocol. This measurement dependency will be addressed in a later section.

In general, paramagnetic materials have the greatest capability for pharmacologic application and can be introduced as soluble, aqueous substances, affording broad flexibility in design and derivation. However, as susceptibility agents, they would not be optimal. On the other hand, superparamagnetic and ferromagnetic particulates are highly efficient because of their extremely large susceptibility and domain structure. Superparamagnetic contrast agents may provide greater applicability than ferromagnetics, even though the latter may possess greater efficiency to induce susceptibility enhancement. Superparamagnetic particles can be made small enough ($< 1 \ \mu m$) to traverse microvasculature and, therefore, can be used as tissue-specific contrast agents. The larger ferromagnetic particles may necessarily be confined to more primary intravascular spaces. In addition, true ferromagnetic substances in vivo could have potential, unforeseen problems associated with their characteristic retention of magnetization.

Relaxation (T1 and T2)

All tissues possess characteristic NMR relaxation properties. *Longitudinal,* or *spin-lattice,* relaxation time (T1) refers to the amount of time it takes for the magnetization to return back to its equilibrium state in the longitudinal direction of the main static magnetic field. More specifically, it is an energy-transfer process between the spins and the environment. Any amount of magnetization that changes from the longitudinal direction to the perpendicular transverse direction by radiofrequency (RF) absorption resides at a higher energy state than at equilibrium. To return to the equilibrium lower-energy level, energy must be transferred from the spins to the environment. Tissues with short T1 values are indicative of high-efficiency rates of energy transfer and faster relaxation back to equilibrium.

Transverse, or *spin-spin,* relaxation time (T2), on the other hand, is a spin-dephasing process that refers to the amount of time that is required for transverse magnetization to lose its spin-phase coherency. This mechanism is based on the molecular environment from spin to spin. The greater the degree of magnetic field inhomogeneity that each individual spin experiences on a molecular level, the more rapid the rate of spin dephasing.

The contrast mechanisms associated with relaxivity are derived from the differences in T1 and T2 of neighboring tissues. Manipulation of contrast based on relaxivity, however, is highly dependent on the method of measurement. In general, measurement parameters can be selected to maximize or minimize the contrast, on the basis of either T1 or T2 differences. An image that demonstrates signal contrast that is based on T1 differences can be acquired by using measurement parameters that maximize T1 and minimize T2 differences. This is termed *T1 weighting.* On the other hand, an image that exhibits signal contrast that is based on T2 differences would be acquired by selecting measurement parameters that maximize T2 and minimize T1 differences. This is called *T2 weighting.*

Contrast enhancement based on relaxivity can therefore be associated with one of two relaxivity processes: T1 or T2. Although the physical basis of T1 and T2 are integrally coupled in their origins, relaxivity contrast agents can be roughly categorized according to the degree of relative change in T1 versus T2. A T1 contrast agent that alters the T1 to at least the extent of T2 is typically referred to as a *positively enhancing* agent, since, in general, it results in a shortening of T1 and an increase in the signal. T2 contrast agents decrease the T2 to a larger degree than T1 and usually are referred to as *negatively enhancing* agents, since they induce faster spin dephasing and more rapid signal loss. In a sense, T2 relaxivity agents produce the same effects as susceptibility agents, but the origins of their contrast mechanisms are different and should not be confused.

The vast majority of contrast media that have been developed and employed in human studies are T1 relaxivity-based enhancement agents. Owing to their large magnetic moments, solubility, and broad flexibility in molecular design and derivation pharmacologically, paramagnetic substances have shown the greatest promise as T1 relaxivity agents. This has allowed the largest degree of freedom in design to develop contrast agents that satisfy most, if not all, of the general requirements previously mentioned.

Motion (Diffusion and Perfusion)

Intensity of signal in MRI is based on the magnitude of the bulk magnetization in the transverse plane that lies perpendicular to the main static magnetic field. Aside from relaxation effects and the method of measurement, this magnetization can be reduced by motion of the spins in the transverse plane. If all the transverse spins are in the same phase of precessional rotation, their collective magnetization is maximized and is referred to as being *coherent* in its phase. Motion during the process of measurement induces spin dephasing or loss of magnetization coherence so that collectively the magnitude of magnetization is effectively decreased, causing a reduction in the signal intensity. Two properties of tissue that lead to this "incoherence" are diffusion and perfusion. Microscopic motions, such as random movement of bulk water in molecular diffusion or the more-ordered movement of blood in microvascular perfusion, can result in signal loss within a voxel of an image. This has been referred to as *intravoxel incoherent motion* (IVIM).[15] Regions of tissue with different degrees of diffusion or perfusion result in contrast by this mechanism.

In theory, selective manipulation of the molecular diffusion coefficient (D) or the amount of perfusion within tissues could be used for the purposes of contrast enhancement. Increases in either would result in a negatively enhancing effect or a decreased signal in the region of enhancement. Diffusion coefficients have been measured and studied at length by MR in spectroscopy[16] and were observed as early as 1954.[17] More recently, this coefficient has been found to have potential clinical relevance in MRI, particularly in neurologic disorders.[15,18] Its specific alteration in the presence of a contrast agent, however, has yet to be investigated.

Actual changes in the degree of perfusion in tissues induced by the presence of an agent have not been studied for enhancement, since such changes would have a physiologic impact. However, enhancement of regions already possessing higher degrees of perfusion and microcirculation by the introduction of agents using other enhancing mechanisms, such as relaxivity or susceptibility, has been preliminarily investigated[8,19,20]. This will be discussed in greater detail later.

THEORETICAL CONSIDERATIONS FOR RELAXIVITY ENHANCEMENT

Since most contrast agent development in MR has been in the area of T1 relaxivity enhancement with paramagnetic materials, it is of interest to describe several of the theoretical considerations associated with the design of a relaxivity agent. Understanding how the T1 and T2 of a tissue are shortened by the presence of a paramagnetic species can provide greater insight into why certain relaxivity contrast agents have been developed. Rigorous theory is beyond the scope of this discussion; however, further reading can be found in a definitive review by Lauffer.[21] Several conceptual overviews have also been presented.[22–24]

The presence of a paramagnetic material affects the T1 and T2 relaxivity of the protons in water. Therefore, the primary aim in the design of a T1 relaxivity agent is to sufficiently shorten T1 without substantially reducing T2 to such an extent that it dominates the relaxation mechanism. Recall that T1 reduction, a positive enhancement mechanism, counters T2 reduction, a negative enhancement mechanism. On the other hand, the aim in the design of a T2 agent is to maximize the reduction of T2. It will be seen that one of the most difficult challenges is to satisfy all criteria for a pharmacologically acceptable agent (e.g., toxicity and stability in vivo), without severely compromising the primary aim of effective T1 or T2 enhancement. In most situations, the goals are counterproductive. Targeting makes the task nearly insurmountable, and highly specific agents have yet to be realized clinically.

Paramagnetism and Relaxivity Enhancement

At the most fundamental level, positive susceptibility is a requirement for relaxivity enhancement, but it is not necessarily sufficient. The existence of unpaired electrons in a contrast agent is paramount to affect T1 and T2 relaxation of water protons. Therefore, diamagnetic substances cannot directly be potential relaxivity agents. Paramagnetic ions have magnetic dipole moments that are typically three orders of magnitude larger than protons. The large local fields of the moments can therefore potentially enhance the relaxation rates of water protons bound to or in the vicinity of the ions. It is the coupled interaction between the ions and the protons that leads to changes in the relaxation.

If, however, susceptibility becomes too large, such as with superparamagnetic or ferromagnetic particles that possess comparatively large domains of unpaired electrons, a much greater influence occurs owing to the significantly larger magnetic moment of the domain or domains. The direct effect of the magnetic moment dominates over the interactive effects between the substance and the protons. This results in a more long-ranged field inhomogeneity, which leads to a shortening of T2 and T2*, that far exceeds any degree of T1 reduction. The material would no longer be classified as a relaxivity enhancement agent, but as a susceptibility agent. Based on first principles of susceptibility,

paramagnetic ions are, therefore, the only plausible choice for the design of a relaxivity-enhancing contrast agent.

Since magnetic moments are directly proportional to the square root of susceptibility, larger susceptibility of an ion leads to a larger magnetic moment and greater interaction between the paramagnetic ion and the water protons. Provided domains do not exist (as in superparamagnetics and ferromagnetics), the paramagnetic ions with the largest susceptibility are, therefore, the ones with the greatest potential as enhancement agents. Many elements in the periodic table are paramagnetic, but the most paramagnetic (highest susceptibility) are first-row transition metals (Mn, Fe, Co, Ni, Cu) and the lanthanides (Eu, Gd, Tb, Dy).

Relaxation Rates, Relaxivity, and Relaxometry

Relaxation times, T1 and T2, are typically discussed in terms of rates. *Relaxation rates* are simply the reciprocal of their respective relaxation times and are additive if they are derived from independent mechanisms. The effective T1 relaxation rate in the presence of a paramagnetic contrast agent, $1/T1_{eff}$, can be expressed as the sum of the T1 relaxation rate of the diamagnetic tissue in absence of the paramagnetic material ($1/T1_d$) and the T1 relaxation rate contribution of the paramagnetic species ($1/T1_p$). Thus,

$$\frac{1}{T1_{eff}} = \frac{1}{T1_d} + \frac{1}{T1_p} \tag{1-1a}$$

The significance of this reciprocal relationship is that the *shortest* T1 contribution dominates the observed T1 relaxation. Similarly, the effective T2 relaxation in the presence of a paramagnetic species follows the same relation,

$$\frac{1}{T2_{eff}} = \frac{1}{T2_d} + \frac{1}{T2_p} \tag{1-1b}$$

and the shortest T2 contribution dominates the effective T2 relaxation.

A further point should be made that $1/T1_p$ and $1/T2_p$ are *contributions* to the observed relaxation rate of the protons by the contrast enhancement agent and do not represent actual relaxations of the paramagnetic species. Intuitively, its extent should be dependent on the number of paramagnetic ions present. For example, if no ions are present, the observed relaxation would simply equal the diamagnetic relaxation of the tissue. In the presence of an agent, the total effective rates can be simply expressed as a linear relationship to the paramagnetic concentration, [M]. As the concentration increases, the contributions of the paramagnetic agent to the total relaxation rate increases. Therefore,

$$\frac{1}{T1_p} = R_1 \cdot [M] \qquad (1\text{--}2a)$$

$$\frac{1}{T2_p} = R_2 \cdot [M] \qquad (1\text{--}2b)$$

where, according to strict terminology, the constants of proportionality, R_1 and R_2, are defined as the T1 and T2 *relaxivity* of the paramagnetic species, respectively. The study and measurement of relaxivity is termed, *relaxometry.* Concentrations are usually expressed as millimolar [mM (mmol/L)] and relaxivity is usually measured as inverse millimolar-seconds (mM^{-1}·s^{-1}). In this manner the interactive effect of a paramagnetic species can be evaluated independently of its concentration in the solution, whether it be in pure water or, for example, in blood.

The foregoing have certain implications that may influence the strategy in the development of contrast agents. Equation 1–1 dictates that the observed relaxation is dependent on the intrinsic relaxation in the absence of a relaxation enhancement agent. In other words, if the intrinsic relaxation rate is slow (i.e., long relaxation time), then the enhancing effect of a paramagnetic agent can be great. Conversely, if the rate is fast, then the effect can be minimal. Equation 1–2 then states that, for the latter situation, it would require a larger concentration to induce the same degree of enhancement as the former and, therefore, require larger doses in vivo.

Compare the effect, for example, of a contrast agent when it interacts with two hypothetically different biological samples having intrinsic T1 relaxation times of 1000 ms and 100 ms. The paramagnetic chelate gadopentetate dimeglumine has a proton T1 relaxivity of approximately 5 mM^{-1}·s^{-1} at 1.5 T.[25] At 0.2-mM concentration, its contribution to the observed relaxation rate is 1 s^{-1}. According to Equation 1–1, the intrinsic T1 of 1000 ms reduces to 500 ms, but the T1 of 100 ms reduces to only 90.9 ms. For the sample with an inherently short T1 to achieve a 50% reduction, a concentration of 2 mM, or a factor of 10 increase in dose, would be necessary. In general, enhancement will preferentially be biased toward tissues with larger T1 values at a given concentration of a contrast agent.

Relaxivity is largely influenced by the external magnetic field strength and thus the Larmor precessional frequencies of protons. In its evaluation, relaxivity is usually measured and plotted over a range of frequencies. This type of relaxivity measurement is termed a *nuclear magnetic relaxation dispersion (NMRD) profile,* and it essentially describes the characteristic enhancement ability of a paramagnetic species. A comprehensive compilation of NMRD profiles and other relaxivity measurements for numerous complexes, free radicals, paramagnetic metal ions, and other paramagnetic species is presented by Koenig and Brown.[25]

The ability of a contrast agent to alter the T1 and T2 relaxation of a tissue depends on its characteristic relaxivities R_1 and R_2, respectively, and its concentration. The chemical and molecular makeup of the agent determine the actual values of R_1 and R_2. The remainder of the theoretical discussion on relaxivity enhancement will conceptually describe the various physical parameters that influence the ultimate relaxivity values. A sound understanding of this is clearly essential to the MR chemist for the development of any relaxivity contrast agent. The brief overview provided here gives those who are interested a better understanding of why some agents are better enhancers than others.

Inner Sphere and Outer Sphere Relaxation

Interactions between a paramagnetic species and the protons of water molecules can be grouped into two distinct categories: inner sphere and outer sphere relaxation. Both can contribute to relaxivity enhancement. They are mutually independent mechanisms and can therefore be uniquely separated into their respective rate contributions to $1/T1_p$ and $1/T2_p$ of Equation 1–1:

$$\left(\frac{1}{T1}\right)_p = \left(\frac{1}{T1}\right)_{inner} + \left(\frac{1}{T1}\right)_{outer} \qquad (1\text{--}3a)$$

$$\left(\frac{1}{T2}\right)_p = \left(\frac{1}{T2}\right)_{inner} + \left(\frac{1}{T2}\right)_{outer} \qquad (1\text{--}3b)$$

If a water molecule binds to the primary, or inner, coordination sphere of a metal ion, then a chemical exchange mechanism occurs between the water and the ion, leading to a contribution to the water proton relaxation rate that is based on magnetic influences and the efficiency of chemical exchange. This is referred to as *inner sphere relaxation.* However, if a water molecule binds to a secondary, or outer, coordination sphere of the ion, or if an unbound water molecule moves within close proximity of the metal ion, then the interactions and effects on the water relaxation rate are considered outer sphere mechanisms contributing to an *outer sphere relaxation.*

In inner sphere relaxation, it would be intuitively clear that there would be a proportionality between its relaxation rate contribution and the total number of water molecules bound to the paramagnetic ion (q). Furthermore, this relaxation would increase if the ion-to-water concentration ratio (p) is increased. A primary goal in the design of paramagnetic contrast agents is to develop agents that allow multiple water molecule-binding opportunities with the inner sphere of the paramagnetic ion. The larger this number, the greater the paramagnetic enhancement by inner sphere mechanisms. Also, the resident lifetime of the water molecule in the bound state (τ_M) plays an important role. Relaxation rates are dynamic by nature, and if the water molecules remain bound for long periods, representing a *slow exchange* process (large τ_M), then the rate of inner sphere relaxation will be slow. Conversely, if *rapid exchange* between bound and free water molecules occurs (small τ_M), relaxation rates will be fast.

Trade-offs inevitably exist when designing a biocompatible pharmaceutical for clinical study. Ideally, use of free metal ions that possess numerous hydrogen-bonding sites would maximize the relaxivity enhancement. However, they are also highly toxic and cannot be used in vivo, even in small concentrations. Therefore, metal and lanthanide complexes have been investigated that increase in vivo stability and reduce overall toxicity. Unfortunately, this will also significantly reduce q and compromise their relaxivity enhancement ability. Other mechanisms can be maximized, however, that still allow substantial relaxivity enhancement even when $q = 1$. Much research has been devoted to this aspect of contrast agent development. Inner sphere contributions to relaxivity vanish if no coordination sites exist for the binding of water molecules to the complex ($q = 0$), leaving only outer sphere effects to enhance the relaxivity.

Inner sphere relaxation is primarily a chemical exchange mechanism between a bound water molecule and the paramagnetic complex that allows electron (ion)–nuclear (proton) interactions to occur in the relaxivity process. Outer sphere relaxation, although less understood and a more complex problem, can be conceptually visualized as an interaction between water molecules and the paramagnetic species, not through chemical exchange of a bound molecular state, but rather through relative translational and rotational diffusion between ions and water molecules in an unbound or loosely bound state. The most generalized description of outer sphere relaxivity also incorporates the effects of fluctuations owing to electronic relaxation of the ion, but is beyond the scope of this discussion.

The effect of molecular diffusion on outer sphere relaxation, at least partially, can be intuitively understood if a hard sphere diffusion model is taken. First, proximity of the metal complex to the water molecule is important. The smaller this distance of closest approach (d), the greater the outer sphere relaxation effect. Furthermore, the faster the translational diffusion motion (τ_D), the better the efficiency of relaxation influence owing to the greater probability of interaction between the metal complex and water. Once again, higher concentrations of the agent will lead to increased relaxivity and T1 shortening in the same fashion as inner sphere relaxation. Keeping small the distance d of closest approach between the ion and water molecule is also important. The cubic geometric contribution of

d is increased by the influence it has on diffusion. The overall influence of d on the relaxation rate in outer sphere relaxation is strengthened to the fifth power. It can also be shown that the greater the environment mobility, the smaller the value of τ_D, which leads to enhanced outer sphere relaxation rates. Large viscosity and large molecules will clearly decrease ion mobility. This leads to less efficient relaxation enhancement by outer sphere mechanisms. Increased temperature will increase mobility and diffusion, thereby increasing the probability for interaction between metal complexes and water molecules and enhancing the relaxivity.

Experimental observations of relaxivity and measurements of $(1/T1)_p$ indicate that outer sphere relaxivity can be significant.[21] Although, in general, the outer sphere contribution is about 10% of the total relaxivity when $q \neq 0$ and inner sphere mechanisms are involved,[26] it nevertheless cannot be ignored in the design of a paramagnetic contrast agent.

Solomon–Bloembergen–Morgan Theory of Relaxation*

The inner sphere contribution to the relaxivity of a paramagnetic species [$(1/T1)_{inner}$ and $(1/T2)_{inner}$] thus far has been discussed in terms of ion-to-water concentration ratio (p) and the number of water molecules bound to the primary coordination sphere (q). Their associated *fundamental magnetic relaxation rates*, $1/T1_m$ and $1/T2_m$, contributed by electron(ion)–proton(water) spin interactions in inner sphere relaxation are based on numerous interactions that occur when the water molecule is bound to the inner sphere of the paramagnetic complex. Since this underlying mechanism dominates the relaxivity of water in the presence of a paramagnetic contrast medium, it has received much theoretical and experimental attention. How to strategically alter T1$_m$ and T2$_m$ currently forms the basis for most research and development of relaxivity contrast agents and warrants discussion. Further description of this theory can be found elsewhere.[21]

In 1948, Bloembergen and colleagues[2] theoretically formulated the relaxation of water protons in the presence of paramagnetic ions. This was refined by Solomon[27] in 1955, which led to the generalized theory of inner sphere relaxation and the so-called Solomon–Bloembergen equations for $1/T1_m$ and $1/T2m$. A further extension of the theory was later incorporated by Bloembergen and Morgan[28] to account for fluctuations in the electronic relaxation time of the paramagnetic unpaired electrons. Inclusion of this has led to the Solomon–

---

*The material in the following seven sections is more technical in nature and may be omitted or scanned by the general reader without loss of chapter continuity.

Bloembergen–Morgan equations, which more completely describe the paramagnetic contribution to proton relaxivity owing to inner sphere interactions.

According to theory, two distinct components of $T1_m$ and $T2_m$ exist, and the relations can be expressed as

$$\frac{1}{T1_m}, \frac{1}{T2_m} = \begin{pmatrix} \text{Dipole–dipole} \\ \text{interaction} \end{pmatrix} + \begin{pmatrix} \text{Scalar} \\ \text{interaction} \end{pmatrix} \quad (1–4)$$

The *dipole–dipole* term describes a distance-related field interaction mechanism between the magnetic dipole of the water proton and the magnetic dipole of the unpaired electron in the paramagnetic ion. This interaction depends on the total electron spin of the ion (S), the distance between the proton and the ion (r), the characteristic time of molecular rotational and translational tumbling of the water–ion unit (τ_R), the lifetime of the chemically bound water molecule (chemical exchange time, τ_M), the electron spin relaxation time (τ_S), and the Larmor precessional frequencies of the proton and electron (ω_I and ω_S, respectively).

The *scalar* term represents an exchange interaction between the electron and proton spins and arises from the chemical bonds that occur between the two. Therefore, it is sometimes referred to as a contact interaction. This term depends on the total electron spin of the ion (S), the lifetime of the chemical binding between ion and water molecule (τ_M), the electron spin relaxation time (τ_S), and the Larmor precessional frequency of the electron (ω_S). It is logical and should be noted that the scalar term is independent of the dipole–dipole distance r and the tumbling time τ_R, since these pertain to spatial and not chemical bond characteristics of the system.

Paramagnetic Ion Spin Dependence

According to theory, relaxivity contributions of a paramagnetic ion are dependent on its spin state as

$$\frac{1}{T1_m}, \frac{1}{T2_m} \propto S(S + 1) \quad (1–5)$$

where S is the spin quantum number of the total electron spin of the paramagnetic ion. This dependence is present in both dipole–dipole and scalar interactions and influences both terms equally.

For the design of a contrast agent, a paramagnetic substance with the highest spin quantum number is therefore desired, provided it does not severely compromise other criteria. If one recalls that the most plausible paramagnetic elements are the first-row transition metals and the lanthanides, given their susceptibility and number of unpaired electrons, the ones that possess comparatively high spin quantum numbers are Fe^{+3} and Mn^{+2} ($S = 5/2$) of the transition metals; and Sm^{+3}, Dy^{+3} ($S = 5/2$), Eu^{+3}, Sm^{+2}, Tb^{+3} ($S = 6/2$), and Gd^{+3}, Eu^{+2} ($S = 7/2$) of the lanthanide metals. These elements have spin numbers that make them potential candidates as relaxivity agents. Even a slight increase in spin from 5/2 to 7/2 can increase relaxivity significantly. From Equation 1–5, the relaxivity would enhance by a factor of 1.8. Interestingly, although nitroxides have very low spin numbers ($S = 1/2$), they possess other characteristics that influence relaxivity and,

therefore, make them potentially useful relaxation enhancement agents, despite their low spin quantum numbers. The question then remains whether this would be enough to accommodate the lack of spin.

Water–Proton and Unpaired Electron Distance Dependence

One of the most influential factors of the dipole–dipole interaction that can potentially dominate the relaxivity is the distance r between the bound water proton and the inner sphere unpaired electron. This influence is not present in scalar interactions. It would seem logical that the closer the two dipoles reside to each other, the stronger their interactions and influence on relaxivity. Geometrically, there is a $1/r^2$ dependence that, in three dimensions, becomes

$$\left(\frac{1}{T1_m}, \frac{1}{T2_m}\right)_{dipole–dipole} \propto \frac{1}{r^6} \quad (1–6)$$

Typically, the average value of r in a paramagnetic complex is approximately 3 to 4 Å. By simply decreasing r from 3.3 to 3.0 Å (9% reduction), the dipole–dipole relaxivity would increase by a factor of 1.77.

One strategy in contrast design that exploits this large dependence is to induce a change in the orientation of the bound water molecules relative to the metal center. In Mn^{+2} complexes, for example, optimizing the orientation can lead to a reduction in the proton–metal ion distance by approximately 0.2 Å, resulting in a 50% increase in relaxivity.[21]

Dipole–Dipole and Spin–Exchange Correlation Times

Aside from the spin number and distance influencing relaxivity, the remaining dependencies that determine $1/T1_m$ and $1/T2_m$ are time-related and are more-complicated, less-intuitive factors. They do, however, impose effects that describe most of the features seen in paramagnetically enhanced relaxivity and are crucial in the design of an optimum contrast agent.

Three primary characteristic times are associated with inner sphere relaxation and the behavior of dipole–dipole and scalar interactions. It will be seen, however, that it is their collective effect, represented by *correlation times*, that directly influences the relaxivity. One of these correlation times (τ_C) is associated with the dipole–dipole term, and another (τ_e) with the scalar term.

First, because chemical binding exists between the protons of water molecules and unpaired electrons of the metal complex, there is a time associated with it that defines *the lifetime of the chemical binding*, τ_M. Chemical binding, in general, is a dynamic process. Continual exchange of the water molecules from a bound to a free state occurs, the influence of which affects the efficiency of relaxation. The τ_M determines how long the water molecules remain in a bound state with the paramagnetic complex. Small values of τ_M indicate a "fast exchange," whereas large τ_M indicates a "slow exchange." The binding of a metal chelate to a protein is one way of altering

τ_M. This time will clearly be associated with both the dipole–dipole term as well as the scalar term. Additionally, it influences the overall inner sphere contribution to relaxation, as described earlier.

A second characteristic time is *the electron spin relaxation time, τ_S*. It is logical that a relaxation mechanism must exist for unpaired electrons in very much the same way that relaxation occurs for protons, since they are dipoles as well. It then follows that this relaxation will have some effect on the electron–proton system and its combined relaxation. The time scale of τ_S, however, is quite different from relaxation times associated with water alone, being on the order of picoseconds (10^{-12} s). τ_S has a well-understood magnetic field dependence. However, chemical influences in altering τ_S are not well known and are still being studied.

The two times τ_M and τ_S are both associated with the unpaired electron and collectively define *the spin–exchange correlation time, τ_e*. Because they are mutually independent actions, their rates are additive, so τ_e is expressed as

$$\frac{1}{\tau_e} = \frac{1}{\tau_S} + \frac{1}{\tau_M} \tag{1–7}$$

The third primary characteristic time that describes the behavior of the proton–electron system is related to the tumbling motion of the entire metal complex–water molecule structure. This is both rotational and translational and is defined as *the characteristic tumbling time, τ_R*. Freely rotating complexes associated with low molecular weights and smaller structures typically have small τ_R values. Conversely, large immobilized complexes associated with high molecular weights have large τ_R values. This, as well, is an action independent of other time-related characteristics and, when combined with the spin–exchange correlation time, the sum defines *the total, or dipole–dipole correlation time, τ_C*, given by the relation

$$\frac{1}{\tau_C} = \frac{1}{\tau_R} + \frac{1}{\tau_e} = \frac{1}{\tau_R} + \left(\frac{1}{\tau_S} + \frac{1}{\tau_M}\right) \tag{1–8}$$

The time τ_e describes dynamic processes associated with the unpaired electron and its chemical binding to the water molecule. It follows then that it represents the time dependence of the scalar term. τ_C, on the other hand, describes the dynamics of the dipole–dipole interaction of the paramagnetic complex–water molecule, which is not only associated with τ_e, but with the tumbling time τ_R as well.

From Equations 7 and 8, it is important to note that it is the inverse of time, or the characteristic rate, that is additive, and not the times themselves. This is similar to relaxation rate additivity and means that the shortest time constant dominates the correlation time. In the design of paramagnetic contrast agents, many strategies are pursued that alter one or more of the time constants, τ_R, τ_S, and τ_M. It must be kept in mind, however, that it is the collective correlation times, τ_e and τ_C, that affect the relaxivity and not the individual time constants. For example, if the correlation time is dominated by a particular time constant because it is extremely short relative to the others, the influence of another that is being altered (pharmacologically in the design of a contrast agent, for instance) will be negligible on the overall correlation time if it remains comparatively long. It will begin to change the relaxivity only when it becomes comparable with or less than the previously dominant characteristic time constant. Correlation times will always reflect the interaction possessing the shortest time characteristic or the fastest dynamic behavior.

Correlation Time Dependence

The dependence of T1$_m$ and T2$_m$ relaxivity on correlation times is not straightforward. Obtaining quantitative theoretical predictions of relaxivity is still very much an active field of research. Many details underlying several areas are topics of debate, and their theory remains unknown. Although a complete understanding would greatly facilitate the search for optimal relaxivity contrast agents, nevertheless, it is still quite possible to pursue strategies based on the known theory that can at least qualitatively predict the trends.

To proceed with describing the complicated dependence of correlation times on relaxivity, it is best to introduce the concept of a "resonance" behavior of 1/T1$_m$ for correlation times. In the strictest sense, a resonance is a physical phenomenon that induces a large effect when certain conditions are met. Nuclear magnetic resonance, itself, is a true resonance phenomenon that has its basis in the quantum mechanical description of discrete energy states of matter. With correlation times, resonance behavior can be applied conceptually, although not exactly.

In general, if τ^* can be introduced as a *resonance correlation time*, then according to the Solomon–Bloembergen formulation, 1/T1$_m$ can very simply be represented entirely by a linear proportionality to τ^*. On the other hand, 1/T2$_m$ is linearly dependent on τ^* as well as the actual correlation time τ. τ^* is a frequency-dependent term, sometimes referred to as a *spectral density*, that is simply the correlation time τ multiplied by a lorentzian weighting function in frequency. More explicitly, τ^*_{AB} can be defined so that the subscript A indicates either the unpaired electron of the paramagnetic ion ($A = S$) or the proton of the bound water molecule ($A = I$), and refers to frequency dependence associated with the respective Larmor precessional frequency. The subscript B refers to either the dipole–dipole correlation time ($B = C$) or the spin–exchange correlation time ($B = e$). Contrary to what may be expected, T1$_m$ and T2$_m$ are *inversely* related to τ and τ^*. However in one sense, this is logical. The slower the actions occurring between the paramagnetic complex and the water molecules (long τ and τ^*), the more time that is allowed for interactions to induce greater relaxivity, thus shortening T1$_m$ and T2$_m$.

Resonance correlation times are frequency dependent. Figure 1–1 shows an example of τ^*_{AB} over a large precessional frequency range for several different correlation times. Precessional frequency, ω_A, is directly proportional to the external magnetic field B, where the constant of proportionality, γ_A, is the gyromagnetic ratio for the nuclear species A (when $A = I$, γ_I is defined for protons, and when $A = S$, γ_S is defined for electrons, where $\omega_S \approx 658 \cdot \omega_I$). Therefore, τ^*_{AB} can similarly be discussed in terms of magnetic field dependence. At sufficiently low frequency or field such that $\omega_A \ll 1/\tau_B$, resonance correlation times are independent of frequency and approximate the actual correlation times. In other words, $\tau^*_{AB} \approx \tau_B$ as seen in Figure 1–1 at a frequency of 1 MHz. However, when $\omega_A \gg 1/\tau_B$, τ^*_{AB} varies *inversely* with correlation time and decreases strongly with increasing frequency, as depicted at

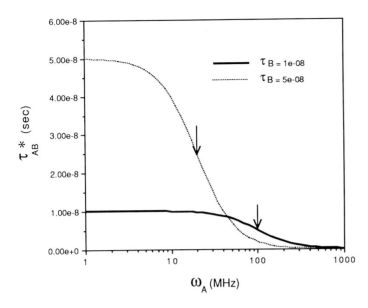

FIGURE 1-1. Dependence of $T1_m$ and $T1_m$ relaxation time on correlation time τ_C at a frequency of 100 MHz. When $\tau_C < 1/\omega$, $T1_m = T2_m$. At $\tau_C = 1/\omega$ (10^{-8} seconds), $T1_m$ becomes a minimum, exhibiting a resonance behavior. As τ_C is increased beyond 10^{-8} seconds, $T1_m$ increases as $T2_m$ continues to decrease.

frequencies above 100 MHz in Figure 1–1. When $\omega_A \sim 1/\tau_B$, τ_{AB}^* exhibits maximum change and a strong dependence on ω_A, beginning with a value of τ_B and decreasing to zero with increasing frequency.

Given the foregoing discussion, the dependence of relaxivity $1/T1_m$ and $1/T2_m$ on correlation time can be more clearly understood. In essence, the behavior of relaxivity at a given frequency is dictated by the behavior of the resonance correlation time at that frequency. A typical situation is demonstrated in Figure 1–2 at a frequency of 100 MHz.

At small correlation times when $\tau_C \ll 1/\omega$ (or equivalently when $\omega \ll 1/\tau$), τ^* approximates τ_C. Since $1/T1_m$ relaxivity is linearly proportional to τ^* and $1/T2_m$ relaxivity is linearly proportional to τ^* and τ_C, $T1_m$ equals $T2_m$, and decreases with increasing correlation time. This is seen in Figure 1–2 when correlation times are on the order of 10^{-10} seconds. At large correlation times when $\tau_C \gg 1/\omega$ (or equivalently when $\omega \gg 1/\tau$), τ^* varies inversely with τ_C. Thus, $T1_m$ now increases with increasing correlation time, but $T2_m$ continues to decrease owing to its explicit dependence on τ_C. This is depicted in Figure 1–2 when τ_C is on the order of 10^{-6} seconds.

Intermediately, when τ_C approximates $1/\omega$ (or equivalently when $\omega \sim 1/\tau$), an inflection, or *resonance effect of relaxivity* occurs for $T1_m$. At precisely the point when τ_C equals $1/\omega$, relaxivity is maximum and $T1_m$ is a minimum. For the situation in Figure 1–2, this occurs when $\tau_C = 1/100$ MHz $= 10^{-8}$ seconds. Correlation times for large metal complexes are typically about 10^{-8} seconds, which puts imaging field strengths in this "resonance" region (1.5 T, for example, corresponds to 63.86 MHz for protons and, thus, $1/63.86$ MHz$^{-1} = 1.6 \times 10^{-8}$ seconds). Not surprisingly, this is close to maximum T1 relaxivity for metal complexes.

The significance of this resonance behavior underscores many strategies in relaxivity contrast agent design when attempting to alter correlation time to enhance the relaxivity. For an optimum positively enhancing T1 agent, the goal is to reduce T1 as much as possible, without producing a situation in which T2 shortening dominates the relaxivity. This condition

occurs when τ_C is altered so that $1/\tau_C$ becomes close to the operating field strength and the corresponding proton Larmor precessional frequency (see Fig. 1–2). On the other hand, the goal in a negatively enhancing T2 agent is to reduce T2 as much as possible. In this situation, pursuing the condition of increasing τ_C so that $1/\tau_C$ becomes lower than the Larmor frequency is advantageous. Generally, design strategies focus on the relationships between correlation times associated with the chemical makeup of the agent and Larmor precessional frequency of the proton associated with the operating magnetic field strength.

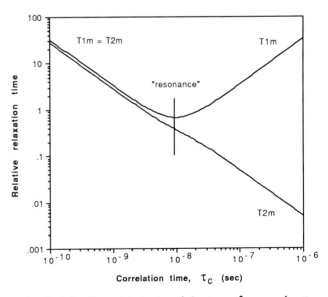

FIGURE 1-2. General behavior of the term τ_{AB}^* as a function of frequency (ω_A) at two different values of correlation time, τ_B. Note that, although the characteristics are the same, maximum change in τ_{AB}^* occurs at 20 MHz when $\tau_B = 5 \cdot 10^{-8}$ seconds, whereas for $\tau_B = 1 \cdot 10^{-8}$ seconds this occurs at 100 MHz *(arrows)*. At low frequencies ($\omega \ll 1/\tau_B$), τ_{AB}^* equals τ_B. At high frequencies ($\omega \gg 1/\tau_B$), τ_{AB}^* approaches zero.

Electron–Spin Relaxation Time Frequency Dependence

The foregoing discussion makes an assumption that holds true under only one condition. It assumes that the actual correlation times, either τ_e or τ_C, are constant over all frequency ranges and field strengths. Of the three characteristic times that define the correlation times, τ_R and τ_M can be assumed to be field independent. However, for τ_S, *the electron–spin relaxation time*, this assumption is not typically true. In fact, it will be seen that it can vary quite significantly with frequency and determines another important resonance phenomenon in the theory of relaxivity. This frequency dependence of τ_S was first formulated by Bloembergen and Morgan.[28]

As described earlier, τ_S defines the electron–spin relaxation time for the unpaired electron of the complex paramagnetic ion and is sometimes referred to as the longitudinal (or T1) electron–spin relaxation time. It needs to be considered only that the type of field or frequency dependence that is exhibited by relaxivity for the bound water would be the same type of dependence experienced by the electron. The type of dynamic behavior specifically characteristic of the electron involves a transient fluctuation of its quantum mechanical spin state that is frequency dependent. It is believed that collisions between the paramagnetic complex and water molecules cause these fluctuations. The correlation time associated with this behavior is defined as τ_V, and the electron–spin relaxivity $1/\tau_S$ can be represented in the same manner as $1/T1_m$ as a linear dependence on resonance correlation times, but based on the Larmor precessional frequency of the electron, ω_S, and the correlation time, τ_V.

Similar to the treatment given for $1/T1_m$ and $1/T2_m$, $1/\tau_S$ exhibits the same dependency on correlation time (here, being τ_V). Qualitatively, at a given field strength (and ω_S), the dependency of τ_S on τ_V is similar to that shown in Figure 1–2 for T1$_m$. Once again a resonance behavior will exist when the precessional frequency of the electron becomes close to or equal to $1/\tau_V$. It will become clear, however, that unlike the design strategies discussed earlier, it is not necessarily true that changing τ_V to match this resonance condition (and thus minimize τ_S) is the correct or only strategy to ultimately minimize T1$_m$. This is clear since there is not a direct dependence of $1/\tau_S$ on $1/T1_m$ but rather an indirect and frequency-dependent effect through its influence on the total correlation time. Furthermore, unlike characteristic times τ_R and τ_M, the theory on how to chemically alter τ_V is not as well understood.

Nuclear Magnetic Resonance Dispersion Profiles and τ_S Influence

The dependence of relaxivity on correlation times for a given frequency has been described. However, to gain the most complete depiction of how correlation times affect relaxivity, NMRD profiles are used in the interest of contrast agent design. The NMRD profiles simply reflect the behavior of relaxivity of a given medium as a function of frequency for correlation times characteristic of the agent.

It can be anticipated that the relaxivity $1/T1_m$ would follow similar behavior to resonance correlation times, since $1/T1_m$ is directly proportional to the resonance correlation times (recall that $1/T2_m$ has an additional dependence on actual correlation times). However, the summation of several of these terms in the relaxivity and the potential dominance on τ_C of the frequency-dependent electron–spin relaxation, τ_S, incorporates several interesting features into the NMRD relaxivity profiles.

Primarily two basic types of NMRD profile behavior exist: one in which correlation times, τ_C and τ_e, *are independent of frequency* (case 1), and the other in which τ_C and τ_e *are dependent on frequency* (case 2). This indicates that case 1 is a situation in which τ_C must be relatively independent of the frequency-varying electron–spin relaxation time and, therefore, means that compared with τ_R and τ_M (frequency-independent parameters), τ_S must be large. In case 2, a frequency dependence of τ_C means that it must be influenced or dominated by τ_S, which in turn indicates that τ_S must be small relative to τ_R and τ_M. In the following NMRD profile descriptions, only relaxivity for dipole–dipole interactions will be discussed for the sake of clarity, although the same behavior is also found as well in the most general situation.

CASE 1 (FREQUENCY-INDEPENDENT τ_C; LARGE τ_S)

Consider the limit when τ_S is large enough compared with τ_R and τ_M that its contribution to τ_C is negligible at all frequencies. Correlation time τ_C will be invariant with frequency at all frequencies. Then $1/T1_m$ and $1/T2_m$ would have a dependence on frequency as shown in the NMRD profile in Figure 1–3. The profile exhibits a characteristic "two-hump" behavior. At low frequency, the first hump is dominated by a τ_{SC}^* term that rapidly falls off to a zero contribution when $\omega_S > 1/\tau_C$ or when $658 \cdot \omega_I > 1/\tau_C$. Note that it exhibits the same behavior as the resonance correlation time as shown in Figure 1–1. As frequency is increased, a second term in the relaxivity, τ_{IC}^*, begins to contribute to the relaxivity until the frequency reaches a value such that $\omega_I \sim 1/\tau_C$. A second hump then occurs. This two-hump characteristic of NMRD profiles simply reflects the summation of two different resonance correlation times. A further increase in frequency makes $1/T1_m$ vanish, but $1/T2_m$ approaches a nonzero constant value dominated by a τ_C term that does not exist for $1/T1_m$. Note that the gradually progressive discrepancy between relaxivities with increasing frequency is due to this linear dependence with τ_C in the $1/T2_m$ relaxivity. Thus, in the design of a T1 relaxivity contrast agent, it is advantageous at higher field strengths to assure that $\omega_I < 1/\tau_C$ when altering τ_C to optimize the agent characteristics.

CASE 2 (FREQUENCY-DEPENDENT τ_C; SMALL τ_S)

In the situation in which τ_C is dependent on frequency, not only does the relaxivity vary with resonance correlation times τ^*, but now τ_C also varies with frequency because of the significance of τ_S. This will depend on the extent of the contribution of τ_S to τ_C. As previously discussed, $1/\tau_S$ is entirely dependent on resonance correlation times, which means that $1/\tau_S$ will follow the dependence with frequency as shown in Figure 1–1. The point at which $1/\tau_S$ falls rapidly to zero will occur when $\omega_S \geq 1/\tau_V$. This indicates that when the frequency is much less than $1/\tau_V$, $1/\tau_S$ is large and τ_S is small. Conversely, when the frequency is much larger than $1/\tau_V$, $1/\tau_S$ is small and τ_S becomes large. Inevitably, if a τ_S dominance of τ_C exists (in cases where τ_R and τ_M are comparably large), it will exist primarily at low frequency, but will vanish at high frequency, and the most rapid change in τ_C with frequency occurs when $\omega_S \sim 1/\tau_V$ (Fig. 1–4). Note that at low frequencies where $\omega_S \ll 1/\tau_V$, τ_C is small and is dominated by τ_S. When $\omega_S \sim 1/\tau_V$, the dominance of τ_S drops rapidly, and τ_C approaches a value dictated by τ_R and τ_M. Finally, when $\omega_S \gg 1/\tau_V$, no influence of τ_S on τ_C exists, and τ_C becomes dependent only on τ_R and τ_M.

This frequency behavior of τ_C must now be coupled with the relaxivity dependence on frequency. Consider Figure 1–3 if it is influenced by the characteristics of Figure 1–4. A typical situation is shown in Figure 1–5. In general, at low frequencies, relaxivity varies with varying τ_C according to the dominance of τ_S. However, τ_C is much smaller when dominated by τ_S at low frequency, as shown in Figure 1–3. Therefore, the relaxivity at low frequency shown in Figure 1–3 now becomes significantly suppressed in Figure 1–5. Depending on the actual values of τ_S, τ_R, and τ_M, and their inverse relationship to ω_I

and ω_S, a dip in the relaxivity could occur when $\omega_S \sim 1/\tau_C$, indicative of the τ_{SC}^* term.

As frequency is increased, the dominance of τ_S vanishes, resulting in a rapid increase in τ_C, shown in Figure 1–4. This causes a resultant increase in relaxivity approximately to the levels indicated in Figure 1–3. When frequency is further increased, the relaxivity drops again and follows the exact behavior of Figure 1–3 when $\omega_I > 1/\tau_C$, and when τ_C becomes independent of frequency. Figure 1–5 shows that this results in an NMRD profile with a distinctive single peak, or resonance which is a direct result of the resonance correlation term τ_{SV}^* that influences $1/\tau_S$ and thus $1/\tau_C$, and the resonance correlation terms τ_{IC}^* and τ_{SC}^* that influence the relaxivity. The prominence of this peak will depend on whether $\omega_I = 1/\tau_C$ coincides with $\omega_S = 1/\tau_V$.

In the development of contrast agents in which large relaxivities are preferable for optimum enhancement, if the paramagnetic complex possesses a small electron–spin relax-

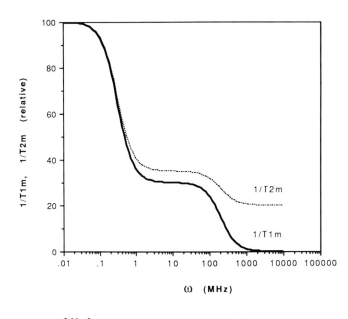

FIGURE 1–3. Nuclear magnetic relaxation dispersion (NMRD) profile of $1/T1_m$ and $1/T2_m$ when correlation time, τ_C, is independent of electron spin relaxation time, τ_S ($\tau_S \gg \tau_R$, τ_M). Deviation between relaxation rates at increasing frequency occurs owing to an additional linear dependency of $1/T2_m$ with correlation time. In this example, $\tau_c = 5 \cdot 10^{-9}$ seconds. A first hump is exhibited when $1/\tau_C$ matches the frequency of the unpaired electron ($\omega_S = 658 \cdot \omega$). A second hump occurs when $1/\tau_C$ matches the frequency of the water proton ($\omega_I = \omega$).

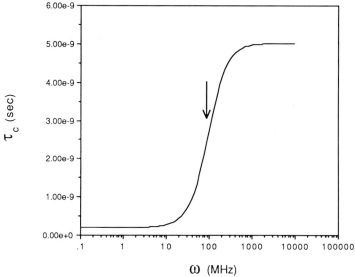

FIGURE 1–4. Frequency dependence of correlation time, τ_C, when influenced by electron spin relaxation time, τ_S. *Arrow* indicates the proton frequency at which maximum change in correlation time occurs. This exists when the inverse of the electron spin correlation time, $1/\tau_V$, matches the frequency of the unpaired electron. At lower frequencies, τ_C is dominated by τ_S, whereas at higher frequencies, τ_C is dominated by τ_R and τ_M.

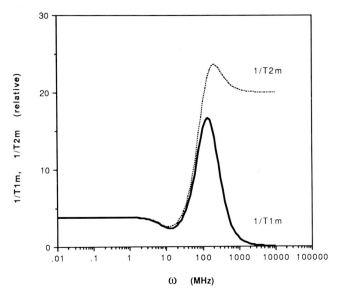

FIGURE 1–5. NMRD profile of $1/T1_m$ and $1/T2_m$ when correlation time, τ_C, is influenced by electron spin relaxation time, τ_S. At lower frequencies, relaxation rates are suppressed owing to the strong dependence of τ_C on τ_S (see Fig. 1–3), whereas at higher frequencies, rate behavior is dominated by τ_R and τ_M. Resonance peaking of relaxation rates occurs because of the increase of τ_C (see Fig. 1–4). At high frequencies, τ_C is independent of frequency and τ_S, and relaxation rates decrease owing to a $1/\omega^2$ frequency-dependence. $1/T1_m$ approaches zero while $1/T2_m$ approaches a finite value because of an additional term of linear dependence with τ_C. Relative scale of relaxation rates is the same as in Figure 1–3.

ation time, it is clearly advantageous to alter the correlation time so that this resonance peak occurs at or near the operating field strength and frequency. In general, however, it is preferable to derive an agent that possesses the characteristics of a large electron–spin relaxation time.

RELAXIVITY CONTRAST AGENTS

On the basis of their susceptibility and, therefore, large magnetic moment, paramagnetic substances have been historically favored for designing relaxivity contrast agents. Transition metals and lanthanides have been chosen for their highest susceptibility (χ). Furthermore, considering the theory briefly discussed in the foregoing, those with the highest spin (S) and most coordination sites (q) provide the largest degree of relaxivity enhancement. Thus, this additionally favors Fe^{+3} and Mn^{+2} ($S = 5/2$) of the first transition metals; and Gd^{+3}, Eu^{+2} ($S = 7/2$), Eu^{+3}, Sm^{+2}, Tb^{+3} ($S = 6/2$), and Sm^{+3}, Dy^{+3} ($S = 5/2$) of the lanthanide metals.

Closer examination of the theory also indicates that large electron–spin relaxation times (τ_S) will lead to less field-dependent relaxivity enhancement and less undesirable reduction of relaxivity at potential operating frequencies (ω_I). Large τ_S would also enable the inverse of the correlation time ($1/\tau_C$) to be in a fre-

quency region more favorable for maximizing overall relaxivity. Because of this reasoning, Gd^{+3}, Mn^{+2}, and Fe^{+3} have historically been considered the optimal choices for starting points in the development of a relaxivity contrast agent.

Much of the search for complexes of ions with various chelating agents has been directed toward maximizing relaxivity, while maintaining low toxicity, high in vivo specificity, stability, and excretability. Discussions of these details and the specific strategies for design and development are beyond the scope of this discussion, but can be found elsewhere.[21,22,24,25,29]

MAGNETIC RESONANCE IMAGING TECHNIQUES WITH THE USE OF CONTRAST AGENTS

The alteration of an NMR parameter by the presence of a contrast agent, whether it is spin density, perfusion, diffusion, susceptibility, or relaxation times T1 and T2, may or may not influence the desired outcome of enhancing the contrast. The types of MRI applications are as numerous as the intrinsic NMR properties of the tissues. Furthermore, each method of measurement, in itself, possesses multiple parameters. Both the type of application and its associated parameters will profoundly affect the contrast attained in the tissues.

Unlike CT, the signal and contrast in MRI are indirect results of the method of measurement and are closely coupled to the NMR properties. Therefore, the selection of the application and measurement parameters can minimize contrast that is related to one tissue characteristic, while maximizing contrast related to another. Inappropriately chosen protocols can, in fact, completely negate the potential contrast-enhancing capabilities of any given contrast agent. On the other hand, enhancement can also be maximized by careful selection of the type of measurement technique.

Since overall contrast is based on the differences of multiple properties of the tissues, the primary aim in the optimization of a protocol when using a contrast agent is to suppress contrast that is based on unchanged tissue properties and to accentuate contrast that is based on the parameter altered by the presence of the agent. It is not obvious, and should be noted, that a protocol with maximum contrast enhancement may not necessarily be considered superior if neighboring tissues exhibit similar signal intensities that hinder detectability. Although a contrast agent may be a T1 relaxation enhancer, for example, the method of measurement with the strongest T1 weighting might be inferior to one that gives slightly less T1 weighting, but clearly better enhanced lesion detectability owing to superior delineation from surrounding tissues. To attain this requires knowledge of the contrast agent enhancing mechanism, the MRI technique, and how measurement parameters are used to alter the contrast, given the NMR properties.

The following is a brief discussion of MRI methods used in conjunction with contrast agents and some of the issues pertaining to the optimization of the protocols. Several papers dealing with this topic, which provide clinical examples, experimental results, and computer simulations, can be found elsewhere in the literature.[23,30–32]

Spin Density

Use of a contrast agent that would alter the regional spin density would require minimizing contrast primarily based on T1 and T2 relaxation, while maximizing the contrast from differences in spin density. In spin echo (SE) techniques, this would entail lengthening repetition time (TR) to reduce T1 contrast, and shortening echo time (TE) to reduce T2 contrast. One disadvantage resulting from this is that imaging time can become prohibitively long, since it is directly proportional to TR. For example, to eliminate the contrast influence of T1 from pure water, TR must be effectively increased beyond 3 seconds. This would result in a scan time of at least 12 minutes with a 256×256 matrix. Furthermore, difficulties are associated with pulse sequences that are designed to provide extremely short TE times (< 10 ms). This may include increased RF power deposition to the patient, increased background noise in the image, and poor slice definition.

Inversion recovery (IR) methods have the additional parameter of inversion time (TI) that primarily manipulates T1-related contrast. Minimization of this would be achieved by shortening TI as much as possible, or increasing it so that the RF inversion pulse preceding the spin echo portion becomes negligible. The latter would offer no advantage. Reducing TI would be feasible, but a large TR would be necessary to completely suppress T1 contrast in a similar way to spin echo, which again would result in long scan times.

Gradient echo (GRE) imaging techniques could provide an alternative that would substantially reduce imaging time as well as RF power. Gradient echo imaging differs from SE and IR methods primarily because of the absence of a 180° RF pulse and the use of RF pulses with flip angles typically less than 90°. Spin density contrast can be achieved by using flip angles of about 10° and TR of approximately several hundred milliseconds. In general, to suppress T1 and T2 weighting in the contrast, the shorter the TR that is used, the smaller the RF flip angle that is required. As well, TE must be kept as short as possible. The major disadvantage of GRE techniques is that the absence of a 180° RF pulse introduces susceptibility into the contrast on the scan and accentuates artifacts associated with magnetic field inhomogeneities. Susceptibility adds a contribution to the T2 spin-dephasing process, and the collective spin dephasing that shortens T2 is referred to as T2*, as previously discussed. Minimizing these effects requires TEs to be even shorter than those used for IR or SE techniques. Inevitably, susceptibility effects will be strong unless TE approaches a zero value, making GRE methods a less than optimum alternative.

Motion (Diffusion and Perfusion)

Imaging to accentuate contrast associated with diffusion or microcirculatory perfusion requires pulse sequences that are specifically designed to be sensitive to microscopic motion. These IVIM sequences employ large gradient pulses, with long durations. Historically, long TE spin echo techniques have been used,[15] and lengthy imaging times have been a main disadvantage. If quantitative data, such as diffusion coefficients, are desired, several long scans are necessary.

One of the primary drawbacks to IVIM spin echo applications is the simultaneous accentuation of bulk motion. Fast-imaging methods[18,33,34] and echo planar techniques[35] have alleviated this problem, but not without a compromise in spatial resolution owing to system hardware limitations.

Although IVIM imaging has received increased interest in recent years, its application with contrast agents that specifically alter diffusion or perfusion characteristics has not been investigated. It should be clarified that, although perfusion imaging with contrast medium has been employed to a large extent in the recent past with dynamic-imaging methods and will be discussed in a later section, the mechanism of contrast enhancement does not pertain to *alterations* in the diffusion coefficients or regional perfusion. Instead, it preferentially enhances regions that already exist, with differentials in the degree of perfusion and vascularity by relaxivity or susceptibility mechanisms of contrast enhancement.

Susceptibility

Susceptibility contrast enhancement necessitates MR techniques that demonstrate T2*, rather than T2, differences in tissues. T2* is a relaxation time that is based on the T2 relaxation of the tissue, as well as additional contributions to the spin-dephasing process resulting from field inhomogeneities and susceptibility. The SE and IR methods use a 180° RF pulse to reverse the spin dephasing that is not related to T2. Therefore, conventional SE and IR techniques are not optimal for susceptibility imaging. Since GRE pulse sequences are absent of the 180° RF pulse, they have been most commonly employed, with an increase in TE causing an increase in T2* contrast and susceptibility weighting.[9,19,36] Modified SE sequences have also been used[8] in which the echo is generated slightly offset in time from the point at which maximum spin rephasing occurs after the 180° RF pulse.

A major drawback of susceptibility imaging, with or without the use of a contrast agent, is the concurrent accentuation of bulk susceptibility artifacts that exist owing to large susceptibility differences at primarily tissue–air interfaces. Efforts have been made to minimize this macroscopic pixel-to-pixel phenomenon by employing high-frequency bandwidth techniques so that susceptibility effects remain microscopically related to only the presence of the contrast medium within a pixel; but the success of these efforts has been limited.

Relaxivity

Since most of the inherent contrast in MRI is dependent on T1 and T2 relaxation, the vast majority of the contrast agent development has been in the area of relaxivity enhancement. A wide variety of potential techniques exist to image the enhancement of relaxivity, and no one technique is necessarily the optimum. Much of the decision depends on the type of situation,[23,30–32] but it is generally essential to choose the appropriate techniques and parameters that will maximize the effect.

Two types of relaxivity contrast agents exist. *Positively enhancing agents* are designed to shorten T1 relaxation as much as possible without reducing T2 relaxation to a larger extent. These, by far, constitute most relaxivity contrast media, in which case techniques that minimize T2- or T2*-related contrast should be chosen. In SE methods, this is attained by using short TR (maximizing T1 contrast) and short TE (minimizing T2 contrast) parameter settings. Inversion recovery is inherently an application that accentuates T1 weighting and may be thought to be advantageous here when employing T1 contrast agents. However, IR may, in fact, possess too much contrast under certain conditions that would make the detectability of an enhanced region more difficult. Moreover, IR techniques are lengthy scans. Therefore, they do not offer a sufficient advantage over T1-weighted SE methods to warrant their general use.

The GRE methods that employ large flip angles, moderately long TR, and that spoil the transverse magnetization can be used, but have the disadvantage of introducing susceptibility artifacts. The one potential use of GRE techniques is in a rapid-scan mode at very short TR (<50 ms) and smaller RF flip angles (~40°), at which T1-weighted images can still be attained in less than 10 seconds. This has advantages in breathhold abdominal imaging and possibly in dynamic-scanning techniques at even shorter repetition times.

Far less developed and clinically used relaxivity

agents are those that shorten T2 relaxation times, thereby dominating the contrast mechanism and are designated as *negatively enhancing agents*. In their employment, T1 weighting is minimized and T2 weighting is maximized. For SE techniques, this necessitates a long TR and long TE, and has the disadvantage of lengthy imaging times. The GRE scans with low RF flip angles can be employed, but once again, exhibit accentuated bulk susceptibility artifacts at tissue–air interfaces.

Because of the dual and coupled nature of relaxation mechanisms, the presence of a contrast agent that alters relaxation inevitably affects T1 and T2 simultaneously. Shortening T1 generally results in a signal increase (positive enhancement), but the reduction in T2 produces an overall signal decrease (negative enhancement). As the concentration of an agent increases, the T1 and T2 relaxation times both decrease according to Equation 1–2. It can be shown that the countering effects of T1 and T2 on signal as a function of concentration result in a well-known concentration dependence that peaks the MRI signal at a given concentration in a given tissue.[30,32] The characteristics of this will heavily depend on the intrinsic T1 or T2 weighting of the type of pulse sequence and the measurement parameters used. Nearly all clinical examinations that employ contrast agents use positive T1 relaxation enhancement mechanisms and a T1-weighted spin echo technique for the protocol. It, therefore, warrants a closer look specifically at the behavior of the MRI signal as it changes with concentration for spin echo techniques.

In general, increasing the concentration of an agent will tend to increase the signal that is based on T1 shortening. Simultaneously, however, increasing the concentration will tend to decrease the signal that is based on T2 shortening. A certain concentration will exist, below which the signal is dominated by T1 shortening, and above which is dominated by T2 shortening. If the implemented pulse sequence is intrinsically T1 weighted (short TR, short TE), the dominance of T1 shortening will occur to a larger extent and over a greater range of contrast agent concentration. On the other hand, if the pulse sequence is T2 weighted, signal intensity will be dominated by T2 shortening over a larger range of concentration, beginning at much smaller concentration levels.

As an illustration of this phenomenon, simulations of signal versus contrast agent concentration are shown in Figure 1–6. The data were obtained at a fixed TR of 300 ms, a value that would accentuate T1 weighting, to demonstrate the signal peaking. The paramagnetic relaxivity contrast agent used in the calculations was gadopentetate dimeglumine (Gd-DTPA). The characteristic relaxivities (R_1 and R_2) were obtained from the literature.[7] Concentrations in millimolar were varied from 0.001 to 100. For comparing the influence of the diamagnetic relaxation times of different tissues ($T1_d$ and $T2_d$), curves were generated for fat (T1 = 260 and T2 = 85 ms) and cerebrospinal fluid (T1 = 2700 ms, T2 = 170 ms). Finally, the MRI signal was obtained from the exact solution of the Bloch equations for a spin echo technique and normalized to a maximum theoretical limit of unity. In addition, fractional signal change was computed. To further illustrate the effects of inappropriately selecting measurement parameters, TE was varied from 10 to 100 ms.

Figures 1–6A and 1–6B show signal intensity and enhancement for fat. Little signal change is seen below 0.1 mM, primarily because of the relatively small T1 and T2 changes at such low concentrations of the contrast agent. Above approximately 0.1-mM concentration, a significant increase in the signal associated with T1 shortening and a positive enhancing effect begins

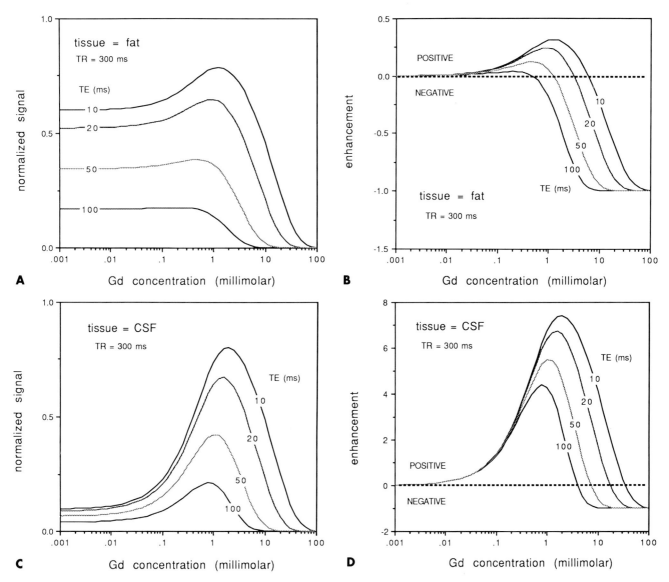

FIGURE 1–6. Simulations of signal and signal enhancement as a function of contrast agent concentration using the spin echo technique. At lower concentrations at which changes in relaxivity are slight, little signal change is seen. As concentration is increased, T1 shortening causes an increase in signal and positive enhancement. When concentration becomes sufficiently large, T2 shortening begins to dominate the signal, causing an eventual negative enhancement. Maximum enhancement occurs at a given concentration that is dependent on the measurement parameters. Overall decrease in positive T1 enhancement as well as a decrease in the concentration that yields maximum enhancement is seen with increasing TE. Intrinsically dissimilar diamagnetic relaxation times of fat **(A, B)** and cerebrospinal fluid **(C, D)** cause significant differences in the concentration sensitivity to the presence of a paramagnetic contrast agent.

to become apparent. Although T2 shortening also occurs, its influence on the signal will depend on the echo time and remains small provided TE is small. In the scenario of strong T1 weighting (TE = 10 ms), maximum positive enhancement does not occur until well above 0.1 mM at concentrations of approximately 1 mM. A further increase in concentration, however, clearly shows a subsequent decrease in signal with domination by T2 shortening. Even at short echo times that minimize T2 weighting in the signal, high-concentration levels with sufficient T2 shortening will result in substantial signal loss. Eventually, enhancement becomes negative even at TE = 10 ms as seen in Figure 1–6B at concentrations greater than 5 mM. Although an increase in echo time will cause peaking of the signal to occur at lower concentration levels, the overall enhancement decreases as TE increases. Therefore, use of the shortest echo times attainable on a given system would be advisable for positive enhancement. On the other hand, if negative enhancement is desired, longer echo times will yield this result at lower concentrations. In Figure 1–6B it is seen that at TE = 100 ms very little positive enhancement occurs at any concentration, whereas negative enhancement begins at approximately 0.5 mM.

The inherent diamagnetic relaxation of a tissue can have a profound effect on the enhancement. Figures 1–6C and 1–6D demonstrate this for cerebrospinal fluid (CSF), which has significantly different relaxation times from fat. Although the peaking of the signal occurs at the same concentration, the degree of enhancement is greatly increased compared with fat, owing to the larger diamagnetic T1 relaxation of CSF. Furthermore, since there is a larger positive enhancement, it requires much higher concentrations to produce a negative enhancement in CSF at any given TE.

Extension of such simulations to clinical applications is not easily accomplished, even if the intravenous administration of the agent is controlled. Tissue uptake of a contrast agent in vivo is dependent on numerous physiologic parameters, such as blood flow, blood volume, mean transit time, and vascular permeability. Ultimately, once an agent has been developed with attractive contrast-enhancing and pharmacologic characteristics, it requires extensive in vivo testing to determine its clinical efficacy. Biodistribution and clearance studies must be performed, along with the investigation of the appropriate measurement technique and parameters before a contrast agent can be completely assessed for its diagnostic usefulness.

The implications of this complex-coupled behavior between concentration and MRI signal are that relaxivity contrast agents require not only careful selection of the pulse sequence type and measurement parameters, but also appropriate choice of administered dose levels and waiting periods so that regional concentra-

tions result in peak signal enhancement. It also implies that relaxivity contrast agents can potentially be used as T1 and T2 enhancers, depending on concentrations and method of measurement. For example, a T1 relaxation agent could, in principle, be used at sufficiently high-dose levels to become T2 relaxation agents under certain measurement conditions. Much of the optimization of MRI applications of T1 contrast agents has been determined to date. However, the use of relaxivity as a dual-enhancing mechanism, either negatively or positively, has yet to be fully exploited. It has been recently studied, for example, that the nonionic gadolinium chelates, such as gadoteridol (Gd HP-DO3A), when administered at doses higher than the presently accepted 0.1 mmol/kg concentration yield improved positive enhancement, indicating that protocols continue to improve and optimum use of relaxivity-enhancing agents has not been reached (Runge VM, Kirsch JE, Thomas GS, 1991, unpublished data).

Dynamic Applications

In recent years, with the advent of subsecond MR techniques, contrast agents have been investigated for their use in dynamic imaging to obtain qualitative and quantitative physiologic information (Dean BL, Lee C, Kirsch JE, et al., 1991, unpublished data).[8,9,19,37,38] Bolus methods similar to those used in xenon-enhanced CT (Xe-CT), single-photon emission CT (SPECT), and positron emission tomography (PET) have shown that MRI has the potential to provide blood flow and other functional information without the use of ionizing radiation.

Two types of contrast mechanisms are currently being used in dynamic MR imaging. Susceptibility contrast imaging techniques offer the most straightforward and simplest opportunity to obtain time–concentration curves necessary to extract pertinent physiologic information.[9,19] By acquiring rapid time-sequential images after controlled bolus administration of a susceptibility agent (1 to 2 seconds per image), region of interest measurements are taken and signal-versus-time data are obtained. Signal decreases are directly associated with presence of the agent (negative enhancement), the degree of which is related to blood flow and blood volume. In principle, the signal can then be directly converted to concentration, based on the exponential behavior between signal and relaxation rate, while assuming the additive relationship between relaxation and concentration. Conventional analysis developed for other imaging modalities could then be employed to extract regional hemodynamic data.

The simple exponential relationship between signal and relaxation rate is possible in dynamic susceptibility imaging because of the independent T2* decay that occurs with echo time in gradient echo techniques. On conventional MRI scanners, the use of a relatively long TE (20 ms) and short TR (35 ms) allows the possibility of obtaining T2*-weighted images in the time resolution necessary for acquiring first-pass perfusion information.[9] This, however, has yet to be accomplished to the degree necessary to extract quantitative blood flow data. By using MRI scanners specially equipped to do echo planar imaging,[37] quantitative information has been obtained.[19]

The second contrast mechanism used in dynamic MR imaging involves T1 shortening and positive enhancement. To date, this has been used in a qualitative manner to obtain information of first-pass perfusion in both the brain (Dean BL, Lee C, Kirsch JE, et al., 1991, unpublished data; Lee C, Dean BL, Kirsch JE, 1991, unpublished data) and in the heart.[39] In these investigations, ultrafast gradient echo techniques (TR < 8 and TE < 4 ms) with the magnetization presaturated by a 180° RF inversion pulse, enable subsecond acquisitions with heavy T1 weighting.[40,41]

Quantitative information about blood flow by this method is less straightforward, owing to the interdependence of the signal with T1 and T2 relaxation. Therefore, a conversion of time–signal curves to time–concentration curves is not as mathematically easy as it is with susceptibility imaging. This is currently under investigation.

SUMMARY

Magnetic resonance imaging differs significantly from CT in that it is a multiparametric-imaging modality both in the intrinsic NMR properties of the tissues and in the methods of measurement. Therefore, the principles of the design and use of MRI contrast agents are multifaceted and will continue to be an area of active research, with many strategies yet to be fully investigated or realized.

The design of an agent must meet the same challenges set forth for any pharmaceutical to be developed for clinical use. In addition, however, the chemistry in altering NMR properties involving spin density, susceptibility, spin, chemical binding, diffusion, molecular structure, and correlation times establishes an entirely different discipline of experimental and theoretical research.

The flexibility to change contrast in MRI adds a further dimension to the use of contrast agents. The concept of negative and positive enhancement is, for example, a common phenomenon in MR. Furthermore, careless manipulation of the measurement techniques can result in completely ineffective contrast enhancement, but it can also enable the identification of the smallest lesions by the introduction of a contrast agent

if techniques are appropriately executed. Although this makes the use of contrast agents in MRI a potentially complicated endeavor, a good understanding of the underlying fundamentals can lead to greater imaging versatility and may result in significantly improved diagnostic efficacy.

REFERENCES

1. Bloch F. Nuclear induction. Phys Rev 1946;70:460–485.
2. Bloembergen N, Purcell EM, Pound RV. Relaxation effects in nuclear magnetic resonance absorption. Phys Rev 1948;73:679–712.
3. Young IR, Hall AS, Bryant DJ, et al. Assessment of brain perfusion with MR imaging. J Comput Assist Tomogr 1988;12:721–727.
4. Wesbey GE, Brasch RC, Goldberg HI, et al. Clinical experience with dilute oral iron solutions used for gastrointestinal contrast enhancement in abdominal NMR imaging. Magn Reson Imaging 1985;3:57–64.
5. Mattrey RF, Hajek P, Baker L, et al. Perfluorohexylbromide (PFHB) as an MRI gastrointestinal contrast agent for proton imaging. In: Proceedings of the fifth annual meeting of the Society of Magnetic Resonance in Medicine. Montreal, Canada 1986, 1986:1516–1517.
6. Saini S, Frankel RB, Stark DD, et al. Magnetism: a primer and review. AJR 1988;150:735–743.
7. Listinsky JJ, Bryant RG. Gastrointestinal contrast agents: a diamagnetic approach. Magn Reson Med 1988;8:285–292.
8. Villringer A, Rosen BR, Belliveau JW, et al. Dynamic imaging with lanthanide chelates in normal brain: contrast due to magnetic susceptibility effects. Magn Reson Med 1988;6:164–174.
9. Edelman RR, Mattle HP, Atkinson DJ, et al. Cerebral blood flow: assessment with dynamic contrast-enhanced T2*-weighted MR imaging at 1.5T. Radiology 1990;176:211–220.
10. Saini S, Stark DD, Hahn PF, et al. Ferrite particles: a superparamagnetic MR contrast agent for the reticuloendothelial system. Radiology 1987;162:211–216.
11. Stark DD, Weissleder R, Elizondo G, et al. Superparamagnetic iron oxide: clinical application as a contrast agent for MR imaging of the liver. Radiology 1988;168:297–302.
12. Renshaw PF, Owen CS, McLauglin AC, et al. Ferromagnetic contrast agents: a new approach. Magn Reson Med 1986;3:217–225.
13. Drayer B. Degenerative brain disorders and brain iron. In: Brant-Zawadzki M, Norman D, eds. MRI of the central nervous system. New York: Raven Press, 1987:123–130.
14. Gomori JM, Grossman RI, Goldberg HI, et al. Intracranial hematomas: imaging at high field MR. Radiology 1985;157:87–93.
15. LeBihan D, Breton E, Lallemand D, et al. MR imaging of intravoxel incoherent motions: application to diffusion and perfusion in neurologic disorders. Radiology 1986;161:401–407.
16. Stejskal EO, Tanner JE. Spin diffusion measurements: spin echoes in the presence of a time-dependent field gradient. J Chem Phys 1965;42:288–292.
17. Carr HY, Purcell EM. Effects of diffusion on free precession in nuclear magnetic resonance experiments. Phys Rev 1954;94:630–638.
18. LeBihan D, Turner R, MacFall J. Effects of intravoxel incoherent motions (IVIM) in steady-state free precessional (SSFP) imaging: application to molecular diffusion imaging. Magn Reson Med 1989;10:324–337.
19. Belliveau JW, Rosen BR, Kantor HL, et al. Functional cerebral imaging by susceptibility-contrast NMR. Magn Reson Med 1990;14:538–546.

20. Young IR, Clarke GJ, Gailes DR, et al. Enhancement of relaxation rate with paramagnetic contrast agents in NMR imaging. Comput Tomogr 1981;5:534–546.

21. Lauffer RB. Paramagnetic metal complexes as water proton relaxation agents for NMR imaging: theory and design. Chem Rev 1987;87:901–927.

22. Engelstad BL, Wolf GL. Contrast agents. In: Stark DD, Bradley WG, eds. Magnetic resonance imaging, St. Louis: CV Mosby Co, 1988:161–181.

23. Gadian DG, Payne JA, Bryant DJ, et al. Gadolinium-DTPA as a contrast agent in MR imaging—theoretical projections and practical observations. J Comput Assist Tomogr 1985;9:242–251.

24. Lauffer RB. Principles of MR imaging contrast agents. In: Edelman RR, Hesselink JR, eds. Clinical magnetic resonance imaging, Philadelphia: WB Saunders Co, 1990:221–236.

25. Koenig SH, Brown RD. Relaxometry of magnetic resonance imaging contrast agents. In: Kressel HY, ed. Magnetic resonance annual 1987, New York: Raven Press, 1987:263–286.

26. Koenig SH, Brown RD. Relaxation of solvent protons by paramagnetic ions and its dependence on magnetic field and chemical environment: implications for NMR imaging. Magn Reson Med 1984;1:478–495.

27. Solomon I. Relaxation processes in a system of two spins. Phys Rev 1955;99:559–565.

28. Bloembergen N, Morgan LO. Proton relaxation times in paramagnetic solutions. Effects of electron spin relaxation. J Chem Phys 1961;34:842–850.

29. Wolf GL, Burnett KR, Goldstein EJ, et al. Contrast agents for magnetic resonance imaging. In: Kressel HY, ed. Magnetic resonance annual 1985. New York: Raven Press, 1985:231–266.

30. Runge VM, Clanton JA, Lukehart CM, et al. Paramagnetic agents for contrast-enhanced NMR imaging: a review. AJR 1983;141:1209–1215.

31. Wolf GL, Joseph PM, Goldstein EJ. Optimal pulsing sequences for MR contrast agents. AJR 1986;147:367–371.

32. Davis PL, Parker DL, Nelson JA, et al. Interactions of paramagnetic contrast agents and the spin echo pulse sequence. Invest Radiol 1988;23:381–388.

33. Merboldt KD, Bruhn H, Frahm J, et al. MRI of "diffusion" in the human brain: new results using a modified CE-FAST sequence. Magn Reson Med 1989;9:423–429.

34. Perman WH, Gado M, Sandstrom JC. DPSF: snapshot flash diffusion/perfusion imaging. In: Proceedings of the ninth annual meeting of the Society of Magnetic Resonance in Medicine. New York 1990, 1990:309.

35. Turner R, LeBihan D. Single-shot diffusion imaging at 2.0 Tesla. J Magn Reson 1990;86:445–452.

36. Edelman RR, Johnson K, Buxton R, et al. MR of hemorrhage: a new approach. AJNR 1986;7:751–756.

37. Dean BL, Lee C, Kirsch JE, et al. Dynamic Gd-DTPA brain imaging and assessment of cerebral hemodynamics with Turbo-Flash imaging. 1990; AJNR (in press).

38. Rosen BR, Belliveau JW, Chien D. Perfusion imaging by nuclear magnetic resonance. Magn Reson Q 1989;5:263–281.

39. Pykett IL, Rzedzian RR. Instant images of the body by magnetic resonance. Magn Reson Med 1987;5:563–571.

40. Lee C, Dean BL, Kirsch JE, et al. A qualitative assessment of patterns of perfusion in cerebral ischemia using ultra-fast MR contrast imaging. 1990; AJNR (in press).

41. Atkinson DJ, Burstein D, Edelman RR. First-pass cardiac perfusion: evaluation with ultrafast MR imaging. Radiology 1990;174:757–762.

42. Haase A, Matthaei D, Bartkowski R, et al. Inversion recovery snapshot Flash MR imaging. J Comput Assist Tomogr 1989;13:1036–1040.

43. Mugler JP, Brookeman JR. Three-dimensional magnetization—prepared rapid gradient-echo imaging (3D MP RAGE). Magn Reson Med 1990;15:152–157.

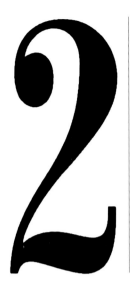

Clinical Applications of Magnetic Resonance Contrast Media in the Head

Val M. Runge

The clinical usefulness of paramagnetic metal ion chelates for contrast enhancement in magnetic resonance imaging (MRI) of the brain is well established. Contrast administration provides both improved sensitivity and specificity of diagnosis in neoplasia, infection, demyelinating disease, infarction, and arteriovenous abnormalities. On the basis of results from prospective studies, use of enhanced scans, in addition to baseline precontrast T1- and T2-weighted scans, is advocated in all patient studies in which there is a high index of suspicion of intracranial lesions. In most centers, use approximates or exceeds 50% of all cases. It is thus appropriate that early developmental work first focused on the use of such agents in brain disease. In the future, paramagnetic agents are likely to play at least as important a role in MRI as comparable iodinated agents do in computed tomography (CT).

OVERVIEW OF CONTRAST AGENTS EMPLOYED IN HEAD MRI

The basic design for this class of contrast agents consists of a paramagnetic metal ion (gadolinium; Gd^{3+}) held rigidly by a chelate. Both linear (DTPA) and cyclic (HP-DO3A, DOTA) chelates have been employed, with the safety of such agents depending primarily upon the strength or stability of the bond between the metal ion and the ligand. Unlike radiographic agents that cause enhancement on the basis of *direct* attenuation, the efficacy of paramagnetic MRI agents depends upon the *indirect* enhancement of relaxation rates and subsequent change in observed signal intensity. The chelate ensures that the metal ion does not react in vivo and is essentially completely excreted. Early research in

1981 and 1982 demonstrated that metal ion chelates could be formulated with sufficiently favorable toxicity and relaxation characteristics for enhancement on MRI, defining the group of paramagnetic metal ion chelates.[1,2] Gadopentetate dimeglumine (Gd-DTPA; Magnevist) was developed as the first agent suitable for human use. Initial clinical trials with gadopentetate dimeglumine were performed in 1983 and 1984, with U.S. Food and Drug Administration (FDA) approval granted in mid-1988.[3–7] In the subsequent three years (1989 to 1991), clinical use grew to dominate head imaging.

Gadopentetate dimeglumine, as formulated for human administration, is an ionic compound; with the –2 charge of the gadopentetate complex being balanced by the presence of two meglumine salts. Although the salt dissociates completely in solution, the safety of the agent itself is dependent upon the stability of the gadopentetate complex. In sharp distinction are more recently developed nonionic agents, such as gadoteridol (Gd-HP-DO3A; ProHance). With the latter agent, the +3 charge of the gadolinium ion is counterbalanced by the presence of three carboxyl groups, each with a –1 charge. Thus, the complex itself is neutral and does not require a cation; such as sodium or meglumine for preparation as an aqueous solution. For all agents (chelates), excretion is primarily by glomerular filtration. With both gadopentetate dimeglumine and gadoteridol, more than 50% of the agent ($t_{1/2}$) is cleared within 100 minutes after administration. Caution is suggested in renally impaired patients. A relative contraindication to use also exists in pregnancy and in lactating women. Gadopentetate dimeglumine is known to cross the placenta and to be present in breast milk[8] in certain species, and the implications to the fetus and newborn have not been established.

For paramagnetic metal ion chelates containing gadolinium, it is the direct coordination and free exchange of water protons with the gadolinium ion ("first-sphere effects") that are primarily responsible for their enhancement characteristics. Relaxation enhancement occurs on the basis of a dipole–dipole mechanism, owing to the presence of seven unpaired electrons on the Gd^{3+} ion. Accordingly, T1 and T2 relaxation times are decreased in the presence of the agent. The effects upon T1 and T2 are competing, with a decrease in T1 producing increased signal intensity and a decrease in T2 producing decreased signal intensity. The result is a nonlinear dependency between the observed signal intensity and contrast concentration. However, at appropriate concentrations, an increase in signal intensity is observed with T1-weighted sequences: thus, "lesion enhancement."

Before one can proceed to interpretation of MR images with contrast enhancement, knowledge of the normal patterns of enhancement is required. With gadolinium chelates, the choroid plexus, pituitary infundibulum, and anterior pituitary exhibit strong enhancement. Venous enhancement is more commonly observed than arterial, although both may be present. Results are dependent on the imaging technique employed, with the use of gradient moment refocusing (GMR) providing a more consistent enhancement of the vascular system. Turbulent and high-velocity flow may, however, remain low in signal intensity. The dura and meninges normally demonstrate a slight increase in signal intensity postcontrast. Pulsation artifacts from both arterial and venous structures remain a pitfall in scan interpretation, often becoming more prominent postcontrast. Comparison of precontrast and postcontrast T1-weighted scans is recommended, considering the difficulty in scan interpretation and the wide range of soft-tissue contrast in MRI. A typical protocol (see the Appendix) would include precontrast T2- and T1-weighted scans, followed by acquisition of postcontrast T1-weighted images, all performed in a single plane. The examination can then be supplemented by T1-weighted images in the orthogonal planes. Spin echo technique is typically employed for visualization of contrast enhancement with gadolinium chelates, although gradient echo technique can also be used. As high-quality fat-suppression sequences become more widely available, their application is likely to increase, owing to the more ready identification of contrast enhancement and differentiation from fat on postcontrast scans performed with such techniques. Fat-suppression sequences are indicated for improved visualization of meningeal disease, soft-tissue abnormalities, and lesions within the orbit. Three-dimensional (3-D) gradient echo techniques show promise for visualization of contrast enhancement on thin (1 to 2 mm) sections with high in-plane resolution.[9] With 3-D magnetization-prepared rapid gradient echo imaging (MP-RAGE), the entire brain can be imaged in less than 5 minutes, with a voxel resolution of $1 \times 1.5 \times 2$ mm (or less). Superior T1 contrast, and thus sensitivity to the presence of paramagnetic contrast media, can be achieved with 3-D gradient echo techniques such as FLASH or MP-RAGE, when compared with spin echo techniques. Sample imaging protocols for the study of brain disease are included in the Appendix.

To some extent the patterns of contrast enhancement observed with intracranial disease on CT scans can be used as a diagnostic guide on MRI (Fig. 2–1). Three primary mechanisms for contrast enhancement exist. An extra-axial lesion can enhance on the basis of (1) intrinsic vascularity. Enhancement of an intra-axial lesion is commonly due to (2) disruption of the blood–brain barrier. Enhancement in arterial and venous malformations is dependent upon (3) the presence of contrast medium in the blood itself, with an additional dependency upon flow rate and turbulence. Although certain types of enhancement are observed on MRI that were not previously described for CT, relative diagnostic specificity can be gained by application of pattern recognition to the enhancement visualized and by classification according to the experience reflected in the scientific literature for both CT and MRI. For example, a meningioma typically exhibits intense uniform enhancement, whereas a garlandlike pattern of enhancement is characteristic for a glioblastoma (see Fig. 2–1). The use of such information does not allow definitive diagnosis, but does lead to improved specificity.

In the interest of time efficiency and patient safety, an intravenous (IV) line is typically placed for contrast administration before the MR scan. Following acquisition of precontrast scans, the contrast medium can be administered through a peripheral port (while closely monitoring the patient). With gadopentetate dimeglumine, administration is typically performed as a slow infusion (1 to 2 minutes for a 15-mL dose). Bolus injection with this agent can cause transient nausea and is not recommended for routine clinical work, particularly because of the close confines of the typical MR scanner. With newer nonionic agents, such as gadoteridol, the lower osmolality allows bolus administration without significant, observed ill effects.

Contrast enhancement on MR imaging of the head results in a change in diagnosis in 3% to 5% of all patients. Additional benefit occurs from increased diagnostic confidence, with improved lesion characterization and, in the event of a negative examination, exclusion of significant abnormality. Adverse reactions with gadopentetate dimeglumine are uncommon, with fewer than 3% of patients reporting pain at the injection site, the most frequently recorded complaint. Anaphylactic-type reactions have been reported, mandating that a physician and appropriate resuscitation equipment be immediately available in the event of a severe untoward reaction.[10]

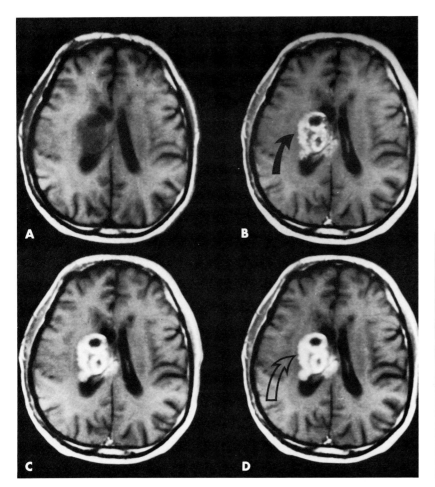
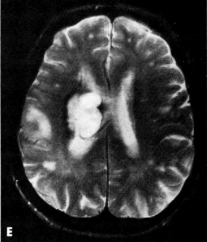

FIGURE 2-1. Grade III astrocytoma. Axial T1-weighted images. **(A)** precontrast and at **(B)** 2, **(C)** 15, and **(D)** 30 minutes post-IV administration of gadoteridol.* **(E)** Precontrast axial T2-weighted image. Enhancement of intraaxial lesions, as illustrated by this patient (*curved arrow,* **B**), occurs with extracellular agents, such as gadopentetate dimeglumine or gadoteridol, because of disruption of the blood–brain barrier. The lesion depicted in this patient lies adjacent to and exerts mass effect upon the right lateral ventricle. With all lesions, a temporal evolution of contrast enhancement occurs. On delayed images, improved enhancement can be demonstrated in some lesions, as here (*open arrow,* **D**), and diffusion of the contrast agent into adjacent tissue may occur. In this specific case, enhancement also permits differentiation, not possible on the T2-weighted examination, of neoplastic disease from white matter ischemic or gliotic changes. (Reprinted with permission from Runge VM, et al. Gd HP-DO3A in clinical MR imaging of the brain. Radiology 1990;177: 393–400.)

CONTRAST USE IN SPECIFIC DISEASE STATES

Neoplasia

Extra-axial

In screening for extra-axial neoplasia, the use of a contrast medium, such as gadopentetate dimeglumine or gadoteridol, is mandated. Both meningiomas and acoustic neuromas typically demonstrate intense enhancement. Meningiomas, in particular, are commonly isointense

*Dosage of contrast medium for all figures was 0.1 mmol/kg unless otherwise stated.

on both T1- and T2-weighted scans (Fig. 2–2), making diagnosis difficult in the absence of contrast enhancement.[11] En plaque lesions, even if hyperintense relative to brain on precontrast T2-weighted scans, are more confidently identified and diagnosed (relative to etiology) on postcontrast scans (Fig. 2–3). Contributing to the lack of sensitivity of unenhanced imaging, in this instance, is the common lack of distortion of surrounding normal anatomy and the absence of other easily recognized secondary findings, such as cerebral edema. Meningiomas that are either hypointense or hyperintense (Fig. 2–4) relative to normal brain on T2-weighted images are commonly encountered, in addition to the isointense lesions just described, with contrast enhancement increasing lesion conspicuity (as

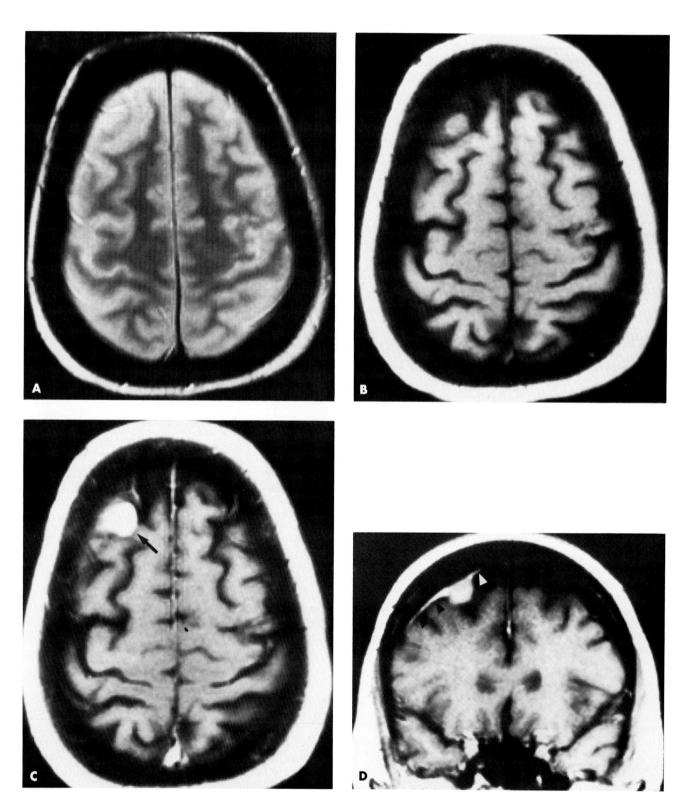

FIGURE 2–2. Right frontal convexity meningioma. Some extra-axial lesions, in particular meningiomas, can be isointense with brain parenchyma on precontrast T1- and T2-weighted images and, thus, difficult to diagnose prospectively without IV contrast administration. Axial **(A, B)** precontrast T2- and T1-weighted, **(C)** postcontrast (gadopentetate dimeglumine) T1-weighted, and coronal **(D)** postcontrast T1-weighted images. Because this meningioma is isointense with adjacent brain and does not cause mass effect, it cannot be identified on precontrast images alone **(A, B)**. The lesion is well seen postcontrast owing to prominent enhancement *(arrow, C)*. Identification of a dural tail *(black and white arrowheads, D)* on the coronal postcontrast image adds specificity to the diagnosis. (Reprinted with permission from Runge VM, Gelblum DY. The role of gadolinium diethylene-triaminepentaacetic acid in the evaluation of the central nervous system. Magn Reson Q 1990;6:85–107.)

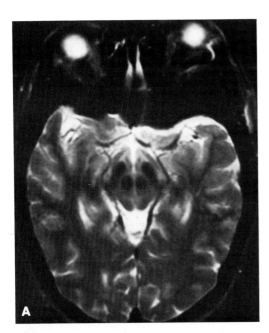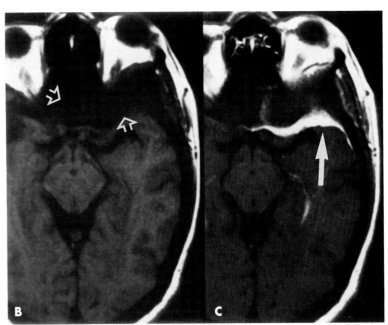

FIGURE 2–3. Left sphenoid wing en plaque meningioma. Axial precontrast T2-weighted **(A)** and pre- and postcontrast (gadoteridol) T1-weighted **(B, C)** images. This meningioma, like that depicted in Figure 2–2, is also not well identified precontrast, primarily because of its en plaque nature, although the lesion is hyperintense to brain on T2-weighted scans. Intense lesion enhancement is seen postcontrast (*arrow*, **C**), making the postcontrast image most efficacious for both lesion identification and demonstration of the full extent of this tumor. En plaque meningiomas represent a common variant in macroscopic appearance and are prone to invade adjacent bone with resulting hyperostosis (also noted here: *open arrows*, **B**). The location (sphenoid wing, extra-axial), dural extent, enhancing characteristics, and adjacent bony hyperostosis lead directly to the diagnosis of a meningioma. This 45-year-old white woman presented with a 2½-year history of visual loss and worsening proptosis. (Reprinted with permission from Runge VM, et al. Clinical safety and efficacy of gadoteridol (Gd HP-DO3A)—a study of 411 patients with suspected intracranial and spinal pathology. Radiology 1991; in press.)

well as providing improved depiction of lesion borders) in these patients. Contrast enhancement permits improved identification of the full extent of the lesion, regardless of precontrast signal intensity characteristics, with plaquelike growth along dural surfaces quite common with meningiomas (Fig. 2–5). Contrast enhancement is also needed for large tumors, to demonstrate the lesion in its entirety. Before the advent of enhanced MRI, diagnostic difficulty was encountered in differentiation of acoustic neuromas and meningiomas occurring at the cerebellopontine angle. Identification of dural extent, as demonstrated in Figure 2–6, enables specific diagnosis of the rarer cerebellopontine angle meningioma. In postsurgical cases (Figs. 2–7 and 2–8), contrast enhancement is needed for identification of tumor recurrence.

In examination of the temporal bone, enhancement on MRI can provide critical diagnostic information. Acoustic neuromas typically demonstrate intense enhancement, with small or large necrotic foci[12,13] not unusual. Lesions that are purely intracanalicular can also be quite difficult to diagnose on unenhanced images alone (Fig. 2–9). The intracanalicular extent of a large lesion is also best recognized following contrast

enhancement (Fig. 2–10). In 225 MR head examinations performed prospectively with gadopentetate dimeglumine at the New England Medical Center, blinded reader interpretation revealed three intracanalicular acoustic neuromas that were diagnosed only on the enhanced examination. The importance of slice thickness for detection of lesions located in the internal auditory canal or at the cerebellopontine angle needs to be emphasized. In a study comparing 5- and 3-mm axial T1-weighted sections, both following contrast enhancement, 22 studies (of 120) were negative on 5-mm sections, requiring 3-mm sections for lesion detection.[14]

Contrast enhancement is mandatory after resection of an acoustic neuroma for identification of residual tumor or recurrence. In a series of ten patients with surgically confirmed residual tumor in the cerebellopontine angle, enhanced MRI provided important additional detail over CT.[15] The investigators also concluded that MRI should be utilized when management decisions might be based on the better definition of tumor detail provided or when multiple follow-up scans were anticipated. Postoperative changes in the brain stem and cerebellum were also better demonstrated by MRI in this patient series.

Extra-axial tumors, specifically including meningiomas and neural-origin tumors, display contrast enhancement owing to increased vascularity.[16] Epidermoid and dermoid tumors do not demonstrate a change in appearance postcontrast. The use of IV agents is strongly recommended in screening patients for extra-axial neoplastic disease. Even with large lesions, which can be readily identified on precontrast scans, the use of enhancement provides improved border definition and assessment of necrosis.

The scientific literature of the early 1980s identified many advantages for MRI (performed without contrast enhancement) over CT. With the clinical introduction of gadopentetate dimeglumine in 1988, the usefulness of MRI in head imaging received a major additional boost, allowing realistic substitution of MRI for CT in the study of most nontraumatic intracranial disease. Scan interpretation has also become more complex; however, diagnostic sensitivity and accuracy have improved. For example, dural spread of a meningioma

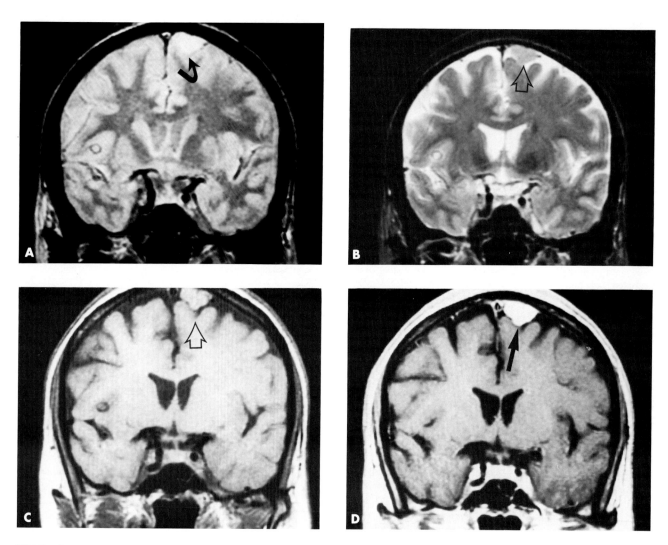

FIGURE 2–4. Convexity meningioma, in a 57-year-old woman presenting with headaches. Coronal precontrast proton density **(A)**, T2-weighted **(B)**, and T1-weighted **(C)** images; **(D)** coronal T1-weighted image following IV administration of gadoteridol. Intense lesion enhancement is observed postcontrast (*arrow,* **D**). This lesion can be identified before contrast administration on the basis of both signal intensity characteristics (hyperintense to brain on the proton density-weighted image: *curved arrow,* **A**) and identification of an extra-axial mass (*open arrows,* **B, C**). Patency of the superior sagittal sinus is confirmed by the presence of a flow void. Meningiomas arise from the dura and do not have a blood–brain barrier. Thus, they typically demonstrate marked enhancement following IV contrast administration. Common locations include the convexity, sphenoid wing, parasellar region, olfactory groove, tentorium, petrous ridge, cerebellopontine angle, and foramen magnum. When present along the cerebral convexity, approximately half are adjacent to the sagittal sinus. (Courtesy of Michael N. Brant-Zawadzki, MD)

was an uncommon finding on CT, primarily because of the difficulty in visualization of soft tissue adjacent to bone. The presence and recognition of such on MRI provides improved diagnostic specificity, advancing the state of medicine beyond that during the heyday of CT.

Intra-axial

Improved depiction of intra-axial tumors following contrast enhancement on MRI occurs by visualization of blood–brain barrier disruption.[17] With astrocytomas, the extent of blood–brain barrier disruption does not correspond completely with tumor extent, for pathologic studies demonstrate strands of tumor cells beyond such borders. Regardless, contrast enhancement, in certain instances, improves tumor versus edema differentiation and permits identification of tumor bulk (Fig. 2–11). As previously noted, enhancement patterns can, in certain cases, improve diagnostic specificity. Typically, low-grade astrocytomas are uniformly hyperintense on

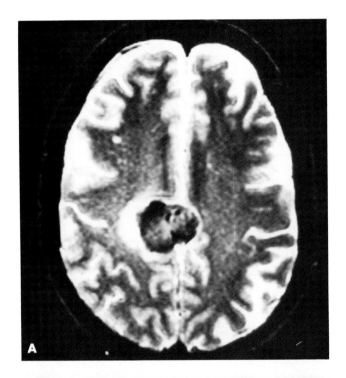

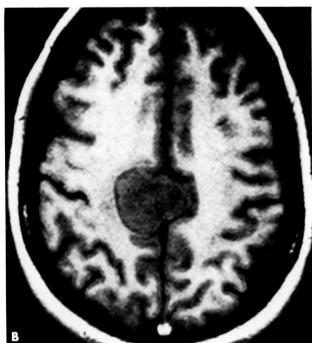

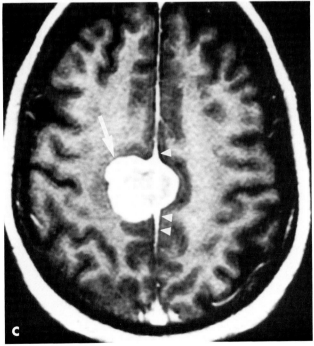

FIGURE 2–5. Falx meningioma in a 65-year-old woman. Axial precontrast **(A)** T2-weighted and **(B)** T1-weighted images; **(C)** axial postgadoteridol T1-weighted image. This meningioma is hypointense on the T2-weighted examination and was calcified on a CT scan (not shown). Signal intensity on T2-weighted images strongly correlates with histopathology. Markedly hypointense lesions demonstrate predominant fibroblastic or transitional elements, as opposed to hyperintense lesions, with predominant syncytial or angioblastic elements. There is intense enhancement of the tumor postcontrast (*arrow,* **C**). The location of the mass (extra-axial, parafalcine) and the presence of an enhancing dural tail (*arrowheads,* **C**) are characteristic for a meningioma. (Courtesy of Steven E. Harms, MD)

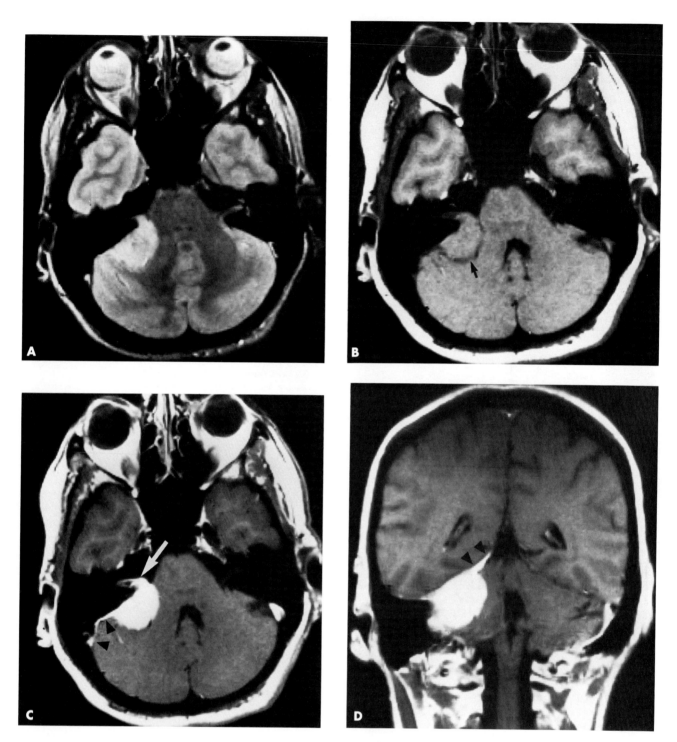

FIGURE 2–6. Cerebellopontine-angle meningioma. **(A)** Precontrast axial T2-weighted, **(B)** precontrast axial T1-weighted, and **(C, D)** postcontrast T1-weighted axial and coronal images. The right cerebellopontine-angle mass is slighted hyperintense on T2-weighted and isointense with brain on T1-weighted precontrast scans. A rim of low-signal intensity can be identified on the precontrast T1-weighted scan (*small black arrow,* **B**), which helps to identify the lesion as extra-axial. Uniformly intense enhancement is demonstrated after administration of gadopentetate dimeglumine **(C, D)**. There is abnormal soft tissue identified both external to and within the internal auditory canal (*white arrow,* **C**). Spread of the lesion along the dura and tentorium (*arrowheads,* **C, D**) can also be identified postcontrast. The latter characteristics, demonstrated only with contrast enhancement, enable characterization of this lesion as a meningioma. Without this information, differentiation from an acoustic neuroma would be difficult. In such cases MRI can provide a more specific diagnosis than CT. This 47-year-old woman presented with right sensorineural hearing loss, with surgical resection subsequently undertaken. (Reprinted with permission from Runge VM, Gelblum DY. The role of gadolinium diethylenetriaminepentaacetic acid in the evaluation of the central nervous system. Mag Reson Q 1990;6:85–107)

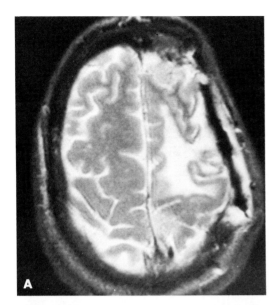

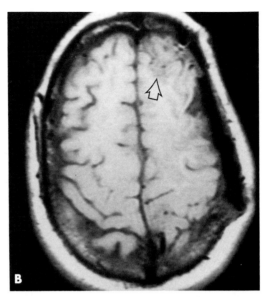

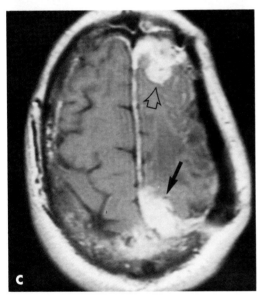

FIGURE 2–7. Recurrent convexity meningioma in a 53-year-old man. Surgical resection was performed 2 years before the present MR examination. Precontrast axial T2-weighted **(A)** and T1-weighted **(B)** images; **(C)** axial postgadoteridol T1-weighted image. Postsurgical changes are noted on the precontrast scans. In the left frontal region, a question of tumor recurrence is raised by the precontrast images, owing to slight hyperintensity on the T2-weighted examination and hypointensity on the T1-weighted examination (*open arrow*, **B**) relative to adjacent brain. The contrast-enhanced scan reveals a large tumor recurrence not only anteriorly (*open arrow*, **C**), but also posteriorly (*arrow*, **C**). This patient was studied as part of a Phase III clinical investigation, with the additional information provided post-contrast (in the opinion of the principal investigator) including lesion detection, number of lesions, improved visualization, disease classification, determination of recurrent tumor, and definition of lesion borders. Postcontrast scans were also felt to provide more diagnostic information than precontrast scans. (Courtesy of Steven J. Pomeranz, MD)

T2-weighted images and do not enhance, whereas glioblastomas demonstrate necrotic regions and contrast enhancement (often intense). However, most intra-axial primary neoplastic lesions (Figs. 2–12 to 2–14) do exhibit enhancement on the basis of blood–brain barrier disruption, with the presence or absence of enhancement aiding little in differentiating histologic types. Contrast enhancement is indicated in planning for stereotactic biopsy, with pathologic studies demonstrating correspondence of blood–brain barrier disruption with higher-grade portions of the lesion. The usefulness of contrast enhancement for lesion detection and delineation of lesion extent in the pediatric population with intracranial neoplasia has also been demonstrated in a limited clinical study.[18] Tumor recurrence, discussed later in depth, is best evaluated by follow-up scans with contrast enhancement (Fig. 2–15). Enhanced MRI performed within 4 days after

resection is advocated for baseline evaluation, with enhancement of postoperative changes being minimal and relatively easily differentiated from residual tumor at this time.[19]

Magnetic resonance imaging is better able than CT to detect pathologic contrast enhancement. Lesion enhancement on MRI depends both upon the concentration of the agent and the intrinsic tissue relaxation parameters. On CT, enhancement is simply proportional to attenuation and, accordingly, to agent concentration, with limitations imposed by beam attenuation. The latter problem leads to poor visualization of enhancement within lesions located in the supraorbital frontal region, temporal lobes, and posterior fossa.

Contrast administration is mandated for the study of metastatic disease. Many metastatic lesions are themselves isointense with surrounding normal brain. In this instance, it is only the presence of surrounding cerebral

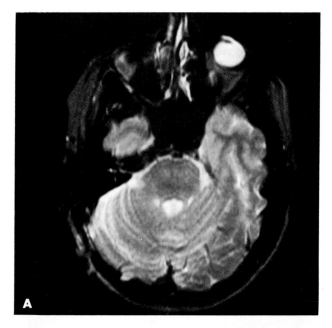

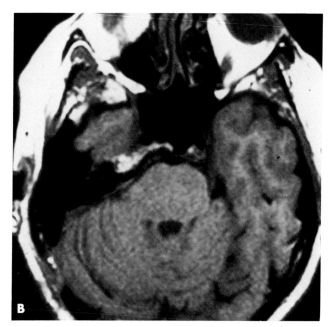

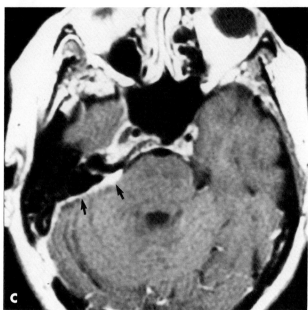

FIGURE 2–8. Residual right cerebellopontine angle meningioma. This 52-year-old woman returned for follow-up MR examination 1 year after resection of a meningioma at the cerebellopontine angle. **(A, B)** Preconstrast T2- and T1-weighted axial images; **(C)** postgadoteridol axial T1-weighted image. Identification of residual tumor (by contrast enhancement on this section and adjacent levels) along the dura and within the internal auditory canal (*arrows*, **C**) was felt by the principal investigator in this study to result in' a change in patient diagnosis. The lesion is unapparent on precontrast images. Caution, however, should be exercised in diagnosis postoperatively of recurrent or residual tumor, which can be mimicked by inflammatory nonneoplastic dural disease. (Courtesy of Burton P. Drayer, MD)

edema that enables recognition on precontrast, T2-weighted scans (Fig. 2–16). Even when the diagnosis of metastatic disease is obvious due to the visualization of multiple lesions on precontrast T2-weighted scans, unenhanced imaging may grossly underestimate the extent of disease (Fig. 2–17). Furthermore, in the absence of secondary findings, including mass effect or edema, small metastatic foci are not commonly identified on precontrast images[20] (Fig. 2–18). Before the introduction of contrast enhancement on MRI, detection of metastatic disease was performed primarily on the basis of T2-weighted images. However, several pitfalls exist, even when such lesions demonstrate differential T2 relaxation characteristics, when compared with those of the surrounding normal brain. For lesions situated peripherally or adjacent to the ventricular system, it may be difficult to differentiate the high-signal intensity of the lesion itself from that of adjacent cerebrospinal fluid (CSF), leading to false-negative scans. Furthermore, small lesions may go unrecognized when adjacent to larger lesions with substantial cerebral edema. The high incidence of ischemic and gliotic white matter changes in the elderly population can further increase the difficulty in identification of metastatic lesions on T2-weighted scans.

The availability of chelates such as gadoteridol, which can be administered at higher doses (>0.1 mmol/kg), is anticipated to further improve detection of metastatic disease by visualization of small and faintly enhancing lesions that otherwise might go un-

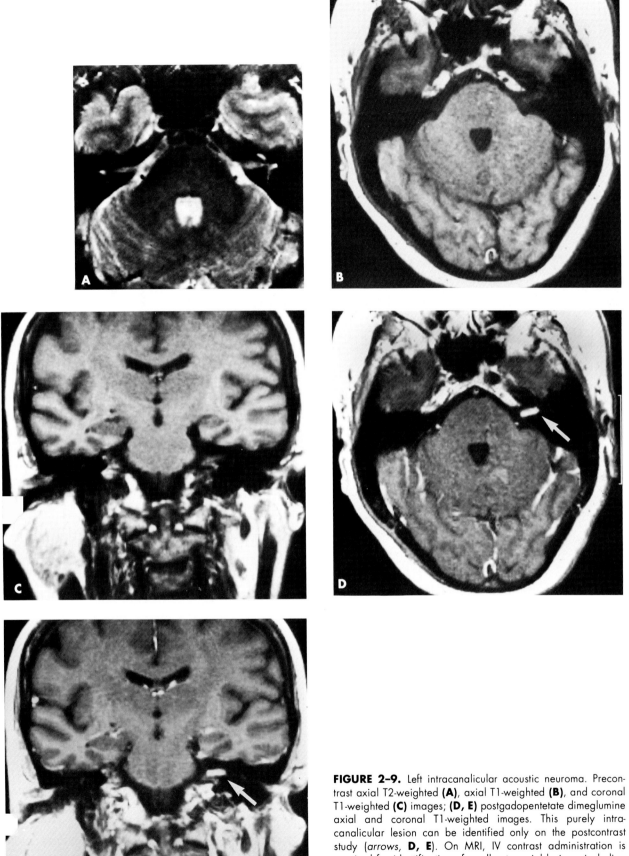

FIGURE 2–9. Left intracanalicular acoustic neuroma. Precontrast axial T2-weighted **(A)**, axial T1-weighted **(B)**, and coronal T1-weighted **(C)** images; **(D, E)** postgadopentetate dimeglumine axial and coronal T1-weighted images. This purely intracanalicular lesion can be identified only on the postcontrast study *(arrows,* **D, E)**. On MRI, IV contrast administration is required for identification of small extra-axial lesions, including acoustic neuromas and meningiomas. (Reprinted with permission from Runge VM, ed. *Clinical magnetic resonance imaging.* Philadelphia: JB Lippincott, 1990)

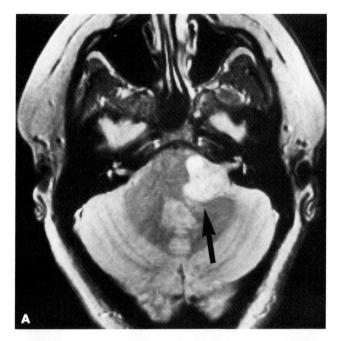

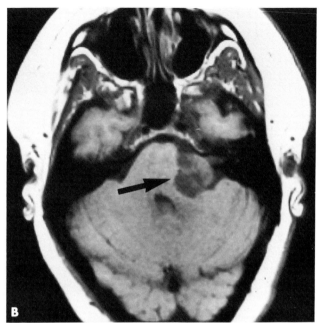

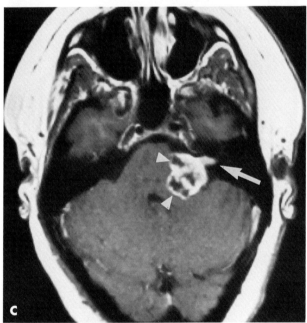

FIGURE 2–10. Left predominantly extracanalicular acoustic neuroma. Precontrast axial T2-weighted **(A)**, and T1-weighted **(B)** images; **(C)** axial T1-weighted scan following gadopentetate dimeglumine administration. On precontrast images, a mass lesion can be identified adjacent to the left internal auditory canal (*black arrows*, **A, B**). There is intense enhancement postcontrast. The intracanalicular extent of the lesion can be identified with certainty only on the postcontrast image (*white arrow*, **C**). Focal nonenhancing regions (*arrowheads*, **C**) within the tumor likely represent necrosis. (Reprinted with permission from Runge VM, ed. Clinical magnetic resonance imaging. Philadelphia: JB Lippincott, 1990)

diagnosed because of partial volume imaging. Such agents would also find application in lesions that demonstrate hyperintensity on precontrast T1-weighted images (Fig. 2–19), with higher administered doses improving the possibility of demonstrating enhancement. Although further conclusions await expanded clinical trials, high-dose contrast administration may also improve the differentiation between benign intracranial and tumoral hematomas by allowing more definite identification of enhancing tumor mass.

Tumor Recurrence

In the follow-up of patients undergoing surgical resection, contrast enhancement on MRI is mandatory for detection of tumor recurrence (Figs. 2–20 and 2–21). The unenhanced examination is not sufficient for detection of recurrent or residual tumor.[21] The use of unenhanced examinations alone in the follow-up of pediatric patients after resection of a brain tumor also cannot be justified. The physician rendering interpretation is obligated to make certain that pediatric referring physicians comprehend the need for contrast enhancement in the evaluation of neoplastic disease, particularly for follow-up, despite the more invasive nature of such study.

Caution is indicated in the diagnostic interpretation of contrast-enhanced scans after tumor resection for two reasons. A study of 32 children with medul-

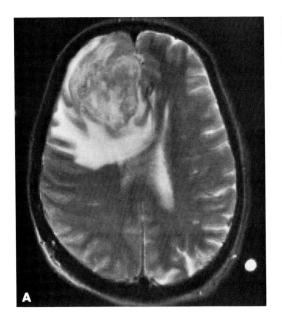
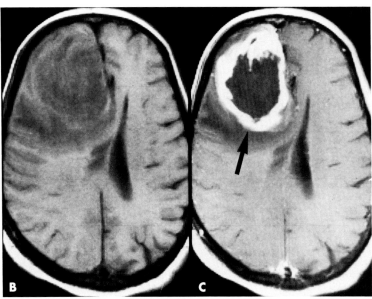

FIGURE 2–11. Grade III astrocytoma. **(A)** Precontrast axial T2-weighted image; **(B, C)** axial T1-weighted images before and immediately after IV administration of 0.3 mmol/kg gadoteridol. The size, location, thickness, and irregularity of the enhancing rim (*arrow,* **C**) and the degree of accompanying cerebral edema are consistent with the diagnosis, which was proved surgically. The identification of tumor necrosis (owing to the lack of enhancement centrally) is possible with certainty only on the postcontrast examination. Note the intense enhancement, in part because of the large administered contrast dose. (Reprinted with permission from Runge VM, et al. Gd HP-DO3A in clinical MR imaging of the brain. Radiology 1990;177:393–400)

loblastoma postoperatively revealed that not all recurrent medulloblastoma tumors enhance.[22] The absence of enhancement with paramagnetic metal ion chelates thus does not definitively indicate the absence of recurrent tumor. Furthermore, enhancement of postsurgical changes can be quite prominent, pointing to the need for early postoperative enhanced MR imaging or demonstration of lesion growth on interval scans taken longer than 6 months after surgery. As with CT, caution is also indicated in the evaluation of patients after radiation therapy. Radiation necrosis can present as an enhancing mass with surrounding cerebral edema and cannot be differentiated by imaging means alone from recurrent tumor.[23] Animal studies have demonstrated that enhancement in radiation necrosis corresponds to a focal region of demyelination. Thus, radiation necrosis on both precontrast and postcontrast images can easily mimic the appearance of recurrent tumor with surrounding cerebral edema.

Diploic Space

Attention must be paid to examination of the diploic space in head MRI so that primary (Fig. 2–22) or metastatic disease (Fig. 2–23) is not overlooked in this location. The marrow present between the outer and inner tables of the skull will appear as high-signal intensity on precontrast T1-weighted scans. Neoplastic lesions and, more specifically, metastases result in marrow replacement, with lesions noted principally as regions of low-signal intensity compared with adjacent high-signal intensity fat on unenhanced T1-weighted images and, at times, as high-signal intensity compared with lower-signal intensity surrounding fat on T2-weighted scans. In certain instances, contrast enhancement can lead to isointensity of a metastatic lesion (which precontrast was of low-signal intensity on T1-weighted scans) in the diploic space relative to surrounding normal marrow. However, enhanced images are superior for detection of small intradiploic metastases.[24] Careful comparison of precontrast and postcontrast images is required. The availability of contrast media that can be administered at higher doses (for example, gadoteridol) as well as imaging with fat-suppression sequences, should further improve diagnosis in the future.

Sellar Region

Pituitary macroadenomas are most commonly isointense with normal brain on both T1- and T2-weighted sequences. However, lesions may appear hypointense or hyperintense on either T1- or T2-weighted images.[25] Pituitary microadenomas commonly can be identified on unenhanced MR images by the slight differences in signal intensity relative to the normal gland. However, in a few cases, such lesions are isointense on both T1- and T2-weighted images. In this setting, only contrast enhancement provides lesion recognition[26,27] (Fig. 2–24). Imaging technique is also

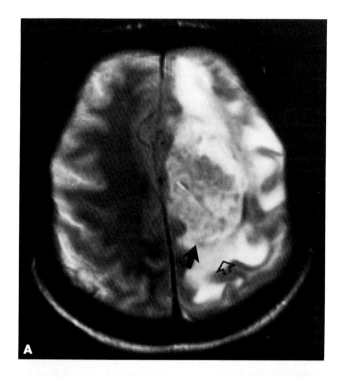

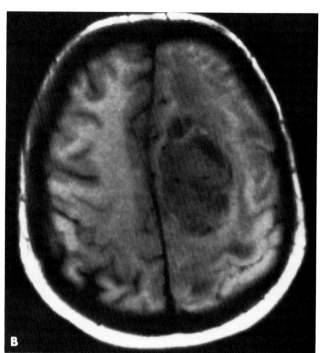

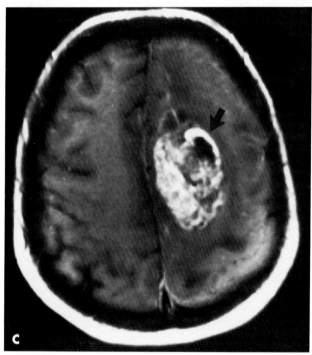

FIGURE 2–12. High-grade ependymoma. Axial precontrast T2-weighted **(A)**, precontrast T1-weighted **(B)**, and postcontrast (gadopentetate dimeglumine) T1-weighted **(C)** images. On the T2-weighted image, the bulk of the tumor mass (*arrow*, **A**) can be differentiated from surrounding cerebral edema (*open arrow*, **A**), although both abnormalities demonstrate a prolongation of T2 (high-signal intensity). Identification of the bulk of the tumor mass (*arrow*, **C**) is improved postcontrast on the basis of lesion enhancement. Caution is indicated, however, in clinical use of such information, since blood–brain barrier disruption (which is visualized by contrast enhancement) may grossly underestimate tumor extent. This 43-year-old woman presented with memory loss and right-sided clumsiness. (Reprinted with permission from Runge VM, Gelblum DY. The role of gadolinium diethylenetriaminepentaacetic acid in the evaluation of the central nervous system. Magn Reson Q 1990;6:85–107)

critical in pituitary studies, with thin sections, high resolution, high contrast, and a high signal-to-noise ratio required. A typical protocol includes initial studies with thin-section sagittal and coronal T1-weighted images. Coronal T2-weighted images and, subsequently, postcontrast T1-weighted images can be employed if the preliminary study fails to reveal a lesion or is insufficient for complete diagnosis. Cavernous sinus inva-

sion can also be more easily discerned on postcontrast studies.

With larger pituitary region lesions, such as macroadenomas (Fig. 2–25) and craniopharyngiomas (Fig. 2–26), contrast enhancement often provides better delineation of the lesion. Characteristic patterns of enhancement in pituitary region lesions (see Fig. 2–26) also improve diagnostic specificity.

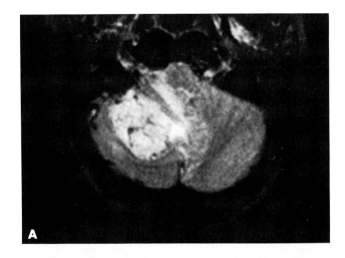

FIGURE 2–13. Hemangioblastoma in a 32-year-old woman, presenting with severe headache and unsteady gait. Axial **(A, B)** precontrast T2- and T1-weighted images; **(C)** axial postgadoteridol T1-weighted image. The portion of the mass visualized demonstrates homogeneous marked contrast enhancement (*open arrow,* **C**), highlighting adjacent abnormal enlarged blood vessels (*black arrows,* **C**). (Courtesy of Ruth Ramsey, MD)

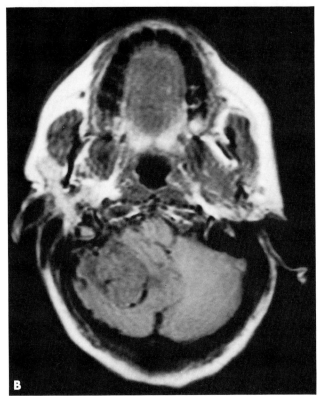

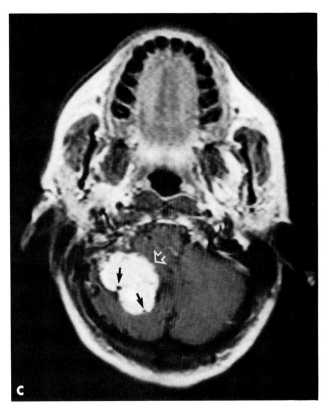

Pineal Region

Germ cell tumors (Fig. 2–27) account for almost all pineal region neoplasms. These arise primarily during childhood, with the most common cell type being a germinoma. Magnetic resonance imaging is an excellent modality for diagnosis, but offers no means for histologic differentiation. Pineoblastoma and pineocytoma are less common lesions, arising from cells of pineal origin.

Infection

The superiority of enhanced MRI over enhanced CT for disease detection was first demonstrated in a canine brain abscess model.[28] This investigation also revealed the superiority of MR studies following contrast enhancement for the detection of parenchymal infection, when compared with unenhanced imaging. Subsequent animal[29] and clinical[30] studies have established the su-

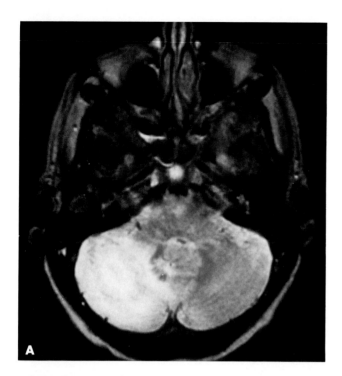
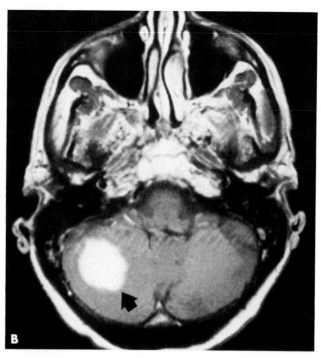

FIGURE 2–14. Lymphoma in a 53-year-old man with acquired immunodeficiency syndrome (AIDS). Axial precontrast T2-weighted **(A)** and postgadoteridol T1-weighted **(B)** images. The postcontrast study reveals a large enhancing mass (*arrow,* **B**) and permits improved definition of lesion border and differentiation of tumor mass from surrounding edema. (Courtesy of Michael A. Mikhael, MD)

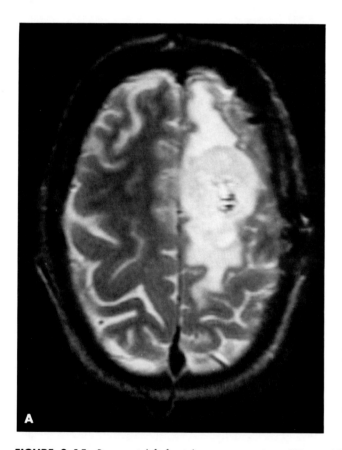
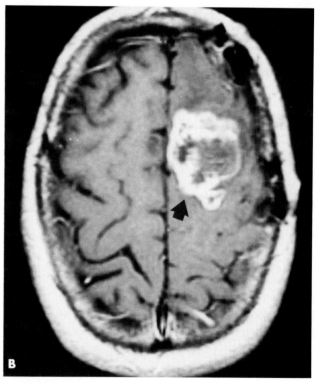

FIGURE 2–15. Recurrent left frontal astrocytoma in a 37-year-old man. Axial precontrast T2-weighted **(A)** and postgadoteridol T1-weighted **(B)** images. There are postoperative changes from a previous left-sided craniotomy. Contrast administration improved the detection of tumor recurrence (on the basis of lesion enhancement: *arrow,* **B**), the distinction of edema from tumor, and resulted in a more definitive diagnosis of recurrent tumor. (Courtesy of Steven E. Joy, MD)

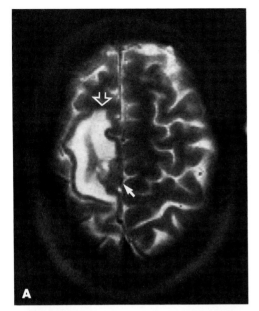

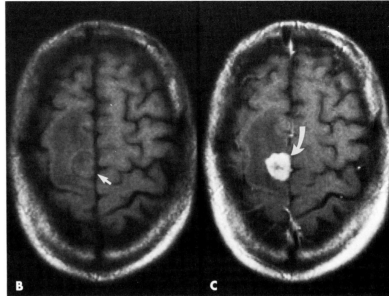

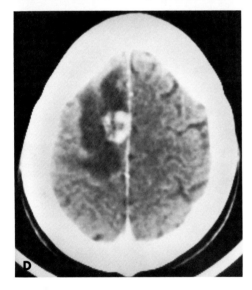

FIGURE 2–16. Right parietal renal-cell carcinoma metastasis. **(A)** Precontrast T2-weighted axial examination; **(B)** precontrast and **(C)** immediate postcontrast (0.3 mmol/kg gadoteridol) T1-weighted axial examinations. **(D)** Postcontrast x-ray CT. On precontrast MR examination, the metastasis itself (*small white arrow,* **A, B**) is difficult to identify because of isointensity with normal brain. Only the presence of accompanying cerebral edema (*open arrow,* **A**) makes diagnosis possible on the precontrast examination. The metastasis demonstrates marked enhancement (*curved arrow,* **C**) postgadoteridol administration. (Reprinted with permission from Runge VM, et al. Gd HP-DO3A in clinical MR imaging of the brain. Radiology 1990;177:393–400)

periority of contrast-enhanced MRI for detection of infection involving the meninges. In a study of 18 patients with meningitis (tuberculosis, bacterial, viral, and fungal),[30] unenhanced MR images were not as specific as either enhanced MRI or postcontrast CT for definition of active meningeal inflammation and focal lesions. With intravenous contrast enhancement, MRI is superior to CT for the evaluation of suspected meningitis. However, precontrast scans are needed for delineation of ischemia, edema, and subacute hemorrhage.

In both the cerebritis and capsular stages of abscess evolution, contrast enhancement can be noted due to disruption of the blood–brain barrier. In the late cerebritis stage, the abscess focus can be differentiated from surrounding edema by contrast enhancement. At this and subsequent stages, ring enhancement is typical (Fig. 2–28). Improved evaluation of disease activity is

also provided by contrast administration (Figs. 2–29 and 2–30). Thus, in the evaluation and follow-up of intraparenchymal infection, contrast enhancement is strongly suggested on MRI.

Bacterial infection of the sinuses can be difficult to diagnose with certainty on MRI, owing to the common occurrence of viral and allergic sinus disease. Enhancement does not provide differentiation, unless secondary changes can be identified, such as meningeal or parenchymal involvement (Fig. 2–31).

Meningeal Disease

Meningeal disease may be the result of neoplasia,[31] surgery,[32] infection, or trauma, with the result on MRI being enhancement postcontrast[33] (Fig. 2–32). Lepto-

(Text continues on page 40)

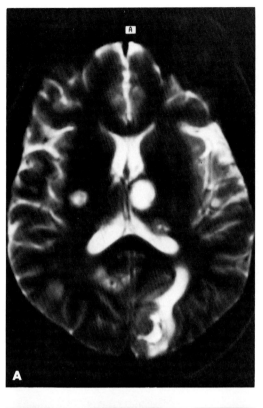

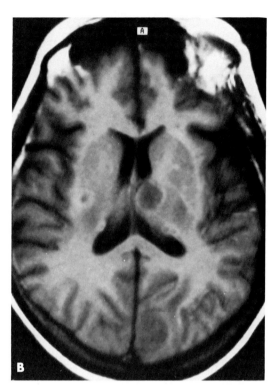

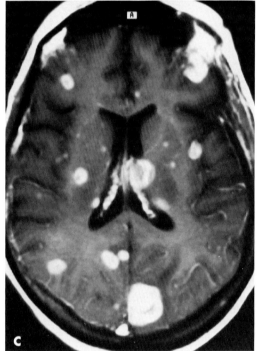

FIGURE 2-17. Metastatic carcinoma of epithelial origin. **(A, B)** Precontrast axial T2- and T1-weighted images; **(C)** axial postcontrast (gadopentetate dimeglumine) T1-weighted image. At least five metastatic lesions can be identified precontrast, primarily on the basis of the T2-weighted examination. Precontrast MRI underestimates the extent of metastatic disease, with more than 20 lesions identified on the postcontrast image. This 55-year-old woman was admitted for evaluation of low back, hip, and knee pain. Metastatic lesions were identified in the lung and bony skeleton, in addition to the involvement demonstrated in the brain. Biopsy of a lower lumbar vertebral body was performed.

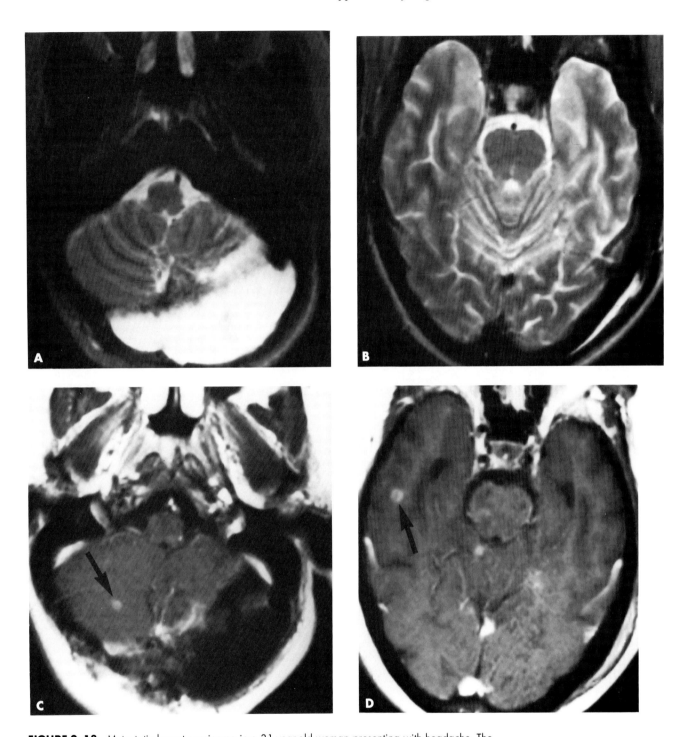

FIGURE 2-18. Metastatic breast carcinoma in a 31-year-old woman presenting with headache. The patient has known metastatic disease to bone and lung. Axial T2-weighted **(A, B)** and post-gadoteridol T1-weighted **(C, D)** sections. Multiple metastatic lesions (*arrows*, **C, D**) on the levels illustrated can be identified only after gadoteridol injection. The lack of accompanying cerebral edema makes prospective identification of these metastatic lesions on precontrast scans difficult. This study was performed as part of a Phase III clinical trial with the postcontrast images judged to be more informative than precontrast images. The additional information gained postcontrast included lesion detection, visualization, disease classification, and number of lesions depicted. (Reprinted with permission from Runge VM, et al. Phase III clinical evaluation of Gd HP-DO3A in head and spine disease. Magn Reson Imaging 1991;1:47–56)

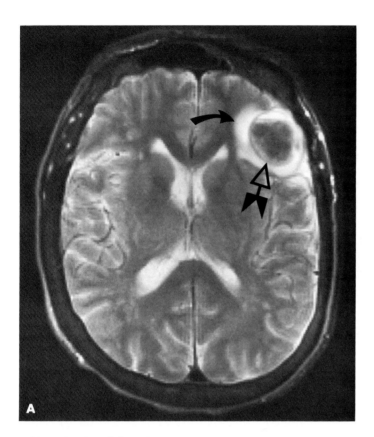

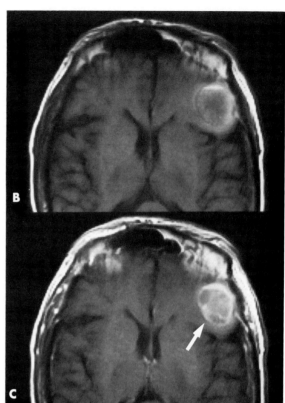

FIGURE 2–19. Left frontal melanoma metastasis. **(A)** Precontrast axial T2-weighted examination, **(B, C)** precontrast and 15-minute postcontrast T1-weighted axial examination using 0.2 mmol/kg gadoteridol. Differentiation of the metastasis (*open black arrow,* **A**) from surrounding cerebral edema (*black curved arrow,* **A**) can be accomplished on the precontrast T2-weighted examination. The metastasis itself is slightly hypointense on T2-weighted examination and slightly hyperintense on precontrast T1-weighted examination, a common finding with melanoma. High-dose (0.2 mmol/kg) gadoteridol administration provides clear identification of contrast enhancement within the lesion (*white arrow,* **C**), a finding that might not have been possible at a lower dose (for example, 0.1 mmol/kg). (Reprinted with permission from Runge VM, et al. Gd HP-DO3A in clinical MR imaging of the brain. Radiology 1990;177:393–400)

meningeal metastases may be diffuse or, less commonly, loculated.[34] Contrast enhancement is important for correct diagnosis and subsequent proper patient management. When a primary soft-tissue mass can be identified, or the meningeal enhancement is nodular, a diagnosis of neoplastic disease can be suggested. Otherwise, it is difficult to determine the etiology of meningeal disease on the basis of MR images alone. Caution is advised in the assessment of disease activity, with dural enhancement observed in some cases for many years after surgery. All patients imaged in the series of Elster and co-workers within 1 year of surgery demonstrated abnormal dural enhancement.[32] Enhancement of the pia mater when found more than 1 year after surgery should be considered abnormal. Brain and meningeal enhancement after intravenous contrast administration at craniotomy sites is more extensive and persists longer on MRI than commonly observed on enhanced CT. Postoperatively, meningeal enhance-

ment may be localized or generalized.[35] Meningeal enhancement postcraniotomy is felt to represent either local inflammation or diffuse chemical arachnoiditis (caused by subarachnoid bleeding at the time of surgery) and does not necessarily indicate either tumor spread or infection. In both infection and after surgery, the depiction of meningeal disease by contrast enhancement on MRI has proved to be superior to that with enhanced CT, with more extensive and persistent disease depicted on MRI. Canine studies have specifically demonstrated the efficacy of enhanced MRI for identification of meningitis, ventriculitis, and cerebritis.[29] The improved depiction of meningeal disease on MRI may be because of comparatively poor visualization on CT due to adjacent bone (and artifacts generated at the interface between the skull and brain). However, improved depiction of ventriculitis and cerebritis may simply be due to the greater innate sensitivity of enhanced MRI to disease processes.

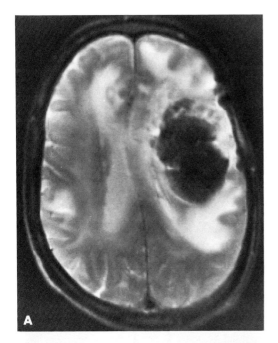

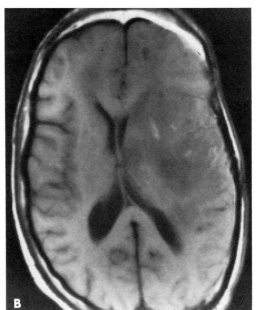

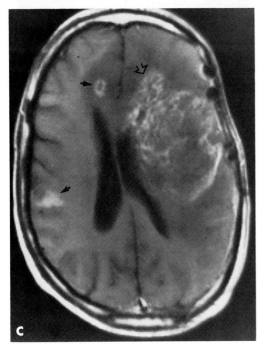

FIGURE 2-20. Recurrent multicentric glioma with large acute, intraparenchymal hemorrhage. Axial precontrast T2-weighted **(A)**, and precontrast and postcontrast (gadopentetate dimeglumine) T1-weighted **(B, C)** images. IV contrast administration is mandatory for identification of recurrent tumor in the brain. In this patient, contrast enhancement identifies tumor bulk anterior to the intracranial hemorrhage (*open arrow,* **C**). However, the lesion is also noted now to be multicentric in origin, with two additional foci demonstrated on the postcontrast examination (*arrows,* **C**). As illustrated by this case, tumor foci may be difficult to identify without IV contrast enhancement when adjacent to larger lesions or in the presence of ischemic white matter disease. (Reprinted with permission from Runge VM, Gelblum DY. The role of gadolinium diethylenetriaminepentaacetic acid in the evaluation of the central nervous system. Magn Reson Q 1990;6:85–107)

Demyelination

Contrast administration enables the assessment of lesion activity in demyelinating diseases (Fig. 2–33).[36,37] In a few cases, lesions can also be identified on the postcontrast scan that are not evident on prospective evaluation of precontrast T1- and T2-weighted images. In an extensive serial study of multiple sclerosis (MS) with MRI, four cases were identified in whom lesions involving the blood–brain barrier (detected only by contrast enhancement) preceded other MRI abnormalities.[38] Contrast enhancement proved critical for lesion identification and provides support for the theory that inflammation and, more specifically, a defect in the blood–brain barrier are early and crucial events in the development of new lesions in multiple sclerosis. Several centers have also employed enhanced MRI to assess disease progression or regression during therapeutic trials. Enhancement on MRI is presumed to be

(Text continues on page 44)

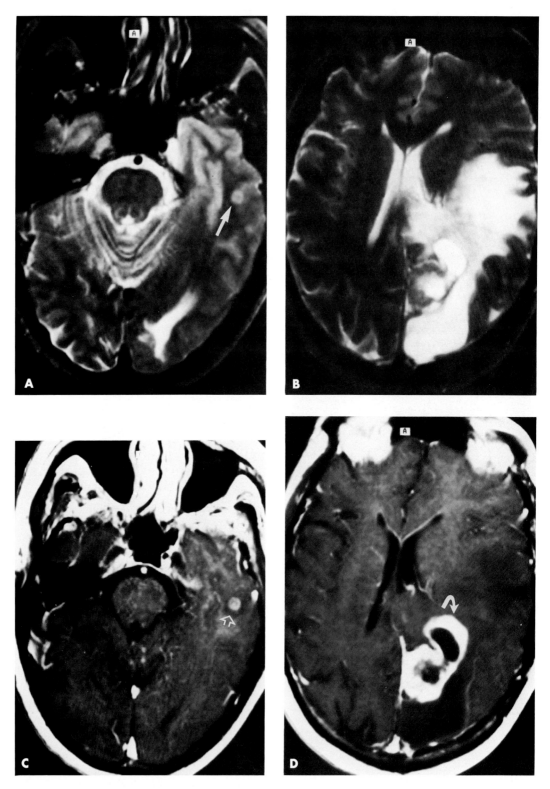

FIGURE 2–21. Recurrent metastatic adenocarcinoma. **(A, B)** Precontrast T2-weighted and **(C, D)** postcontrast (gadopentetate dimeglumine) T1-weighted axial images at two levels. Approximately 3 months before this examination, the patient underwent surgery for gross total excision of the left parieto-occipital metastasis. On the present examination, definitive diagnosis of tumor recurrence in the surgical bed (*white curved arrow,* **D**) and a second metastatic lesion in the left temporal lobe (*open arrow,* **C**) is made possible by contrast enhancement. The small metastatic focus in the temporal lobe can be identified in retrospect on the T2-weighted examination (*white arrow,* **A**), but this lesion does not elicit substantial cerebral edema. Contrast administration is mandated for diagnosis of both recurrent tumor and secondary lesions.

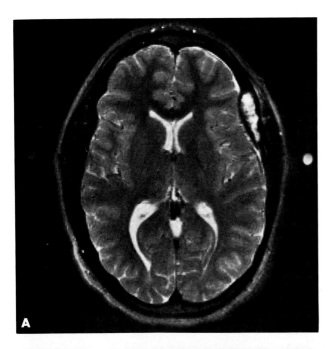

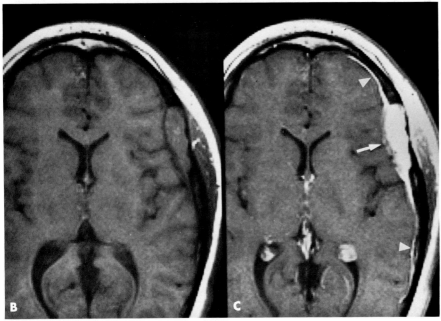

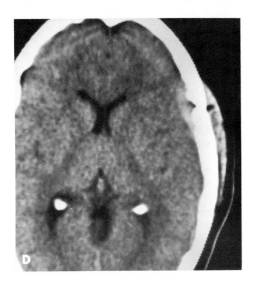

FIGURE 2–22. Eosinophilic granuloma. Axial **(A)** precontrast T2-weighted examination; axial **(B)** precontrast and **(C)** 2-minute postcontrast T1-weighted examinations using a dose of 0.2 mmol/kg gadoteridol; **(D)** unenhanced CT. Marked enhancement of both the bulk of the lesion (*arrow*, **C**) and adjacent meningeal disease (*arrowheads*, **C**) was noted on MRI. The lesion is poorly depicted by CT, with enhancement of the meninges not appreciated on postcontrast scans (image not shown) presumably owing to close approximation of this abnormal soft tissue to the skull.

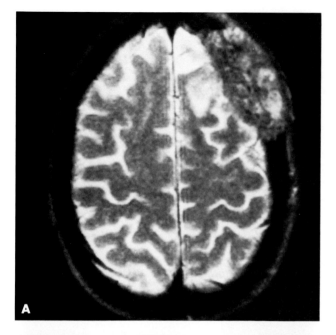

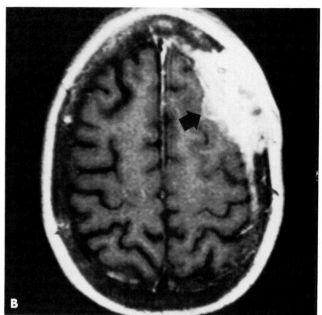

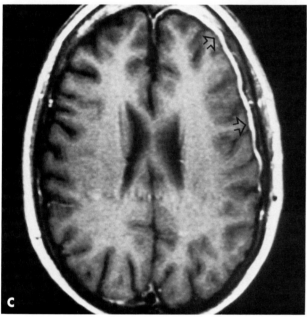

FIGURE 2-23. Adenocarcinoma of the lung metastatic to the skull. This 69-year-old white woman presented with left skull pain 1 month after diagnosis of lung cancer. Axial **(A)** precontrast T2-weighted and **(B, C)** postgadoteridol T1-weighted images. IV contrast administration improves visualization of the main bulk of this skull metastasis (*arrow*, **B**). Involvement of the leptomeninges (*open arrows*, **C**) was recognized only on postcontrast images. (Courtesy of Frank W. Morgan, MD)

a transient phenomenon caused by temporary local blood–brain barrier disruption.[39] Contrast-enhanced studies are more sensitive than unenhanced MRI for the detection of disease activity in multiple sclerosis. A recent study has demonstrated that MRI makes possible improved quantitation of the defect in the blood–brain barrier, leading potentially to information concerning pathogenesis and making possible improved methods for monitoring treatment efficacy in this disease.[40]

Lesion enhancement has been observed in patients with postinfectious encephalomyelitis. Theoretically, enhancement could provide differentiation between this disease and MS. In MS, it is the minority of lesions that will enhance. This should permit differentiation from acute encephalomyelitis, which is a monotonic illness with all lesions of approximately the same age and, thus, the same enhancement characteristics.

In the spinal cord, MS plaques also enhance,[41] presumably reflecting active disease. Care should be exercised in the differentiation of such lesions, which can demonstrate a striking mass effect, from cord astrocytomas.

(Text continues on page 50)

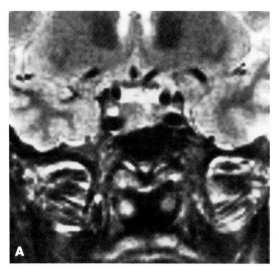
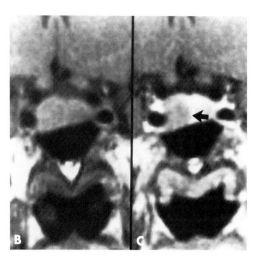

FIGURE 2-24. Prolactinoma. Coronal T2-weighted **(A)** and pre- and postcontrast (gadopentetate dimeglumine) T1-weighted **(B, C)** images. A large microadenoma can be identified on only the postcontrast image, in the right half of the gland (*black arrow,* **C**). There is differential enhancement of the normal and pathologic pituitary tissue, making lesion detection possible postcontrast, with the adenoma demonstrating less intense enhancement on the immediate postcontrast scan. Although most pituitary microadenomas can be identified on precontrast T1-weighted images, the addition of postcontrast scans improves sensitivity. The normal pituitary enhances prominently following IV gadolinium chelate administration. Microadenomas can demonstrate enhancement either greater or less in magnitude, compared with the normal pituitary, with the degree of enhancement dependent, in part, on the timing of the scan postcontrast. (Reprinted with permission from Runge VM, Gelblum DY. The role of gadolinium diethylenetriaminepentaacetic acid in the evaluation of the central nervous system. Magn Reson Q 1990;6:85–107)

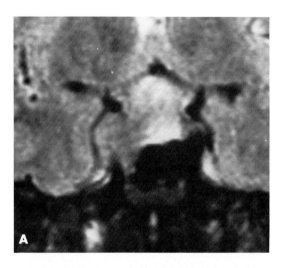
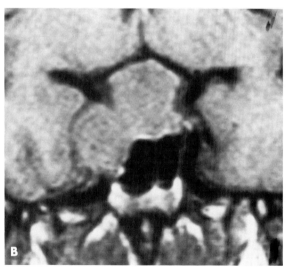
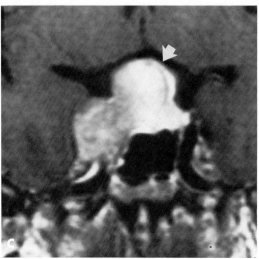

FIGURE 2-25. Pituitary macroadenoma in a 36-year-old woman who presented 4 years before the present examination with galactorrhea, amenorrhea, and elevated prolactin levels. Symptoms progressed to include visual field defects. Precontrast coronal T2-weighted **(A)** and T1-weighted **(B)** images; **(C)** coronal post-gadoteridol T1-weighted image. The lesion is principally isointense with brain on both T1- and T2-weighted images precontrast. This finding, together with enhancement postcontrast (*arrow,* **C**) is characteristic of many pituitary macroadenomas. Contrast enhancement can also improve the ability to assess cavernous sinus invasion, by demonstration of differential enhancement of tumor, compared with venous blood within the sinus. In this patient, the tumor extends laterally to the right without demonstration of normal sinus, suggesting invasion on the right. The study was performed as part of a Phase III clinical trial, with the principal investigator assessing that contrast administration provided both improved lesion visualization and definition of lesion borders. (Courtesy of Frank W. Morgan, MD)

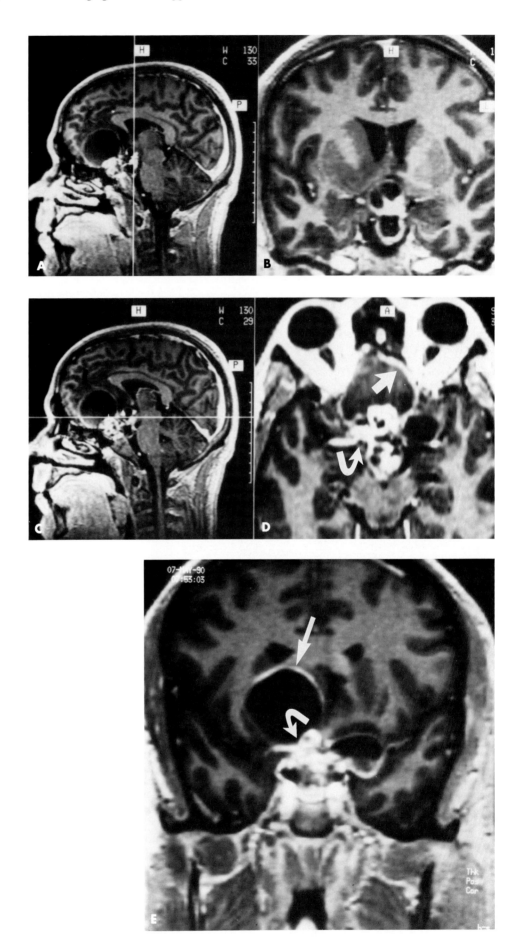

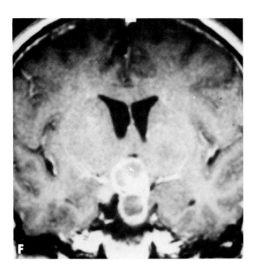

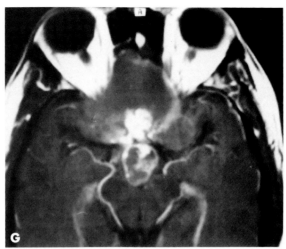

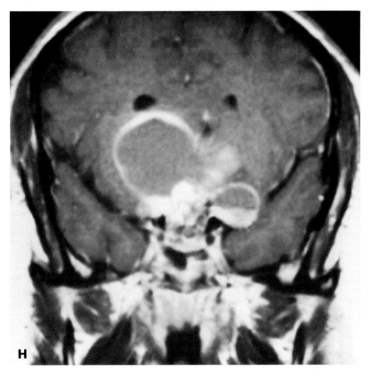

FIGURE 2-26. Craniopharyngioma. **(A–E)** Postcontrast (gadopentetate dimeglumine) reformatted T1-weighted images (1- to 2-mm slice thickness) from a 3-D MP-RAGE examination (5-minute scan time). The vertical line on **A** and the horizontal line on **C** indicate the position for the corresponding coronal and axial sections displayed in **B** and **D**, respectively. **(F–H)** Postcontrast T1-weighted spin echo (5- to 7-mm slice thickness) images (from three separate acquisitions) corresponding in position to the 3-D MP-RAGE reformatted images **(B, D, E)**. Both rim (*white arrows*, **D, E**) and small nodular enhancement (*curved white arrows*, **D, E**) are noted in this primarily cystic lesion, characteristic features for a craniopharyngioma. Enhancement of the rim is best identified on the thin (1- to 2-mm) 3-D reformats. Partial volume imaging on thicker sections, such as that obtained on routine spin echo examinations, can result in nonvisualization of lesion enhancement. The bulk of the lesion was markedly hyperintense on the T2-weighted examination (not shown). This 28-year-old woman presented with a 2-month history of complete vision loss in the right eye and progressive loss of peripheral vision in the left eye. There were associated headaches of progressive severity. Gross total excision of this craniopharyngioma was achieved by a right craniotomy. (Reprinted with permission from Runge VM, et al. Clinical comparison of 3-D MP-RAGE and FLASH techniques for MR imaging of the head. JMRI 1991;1:493–500)

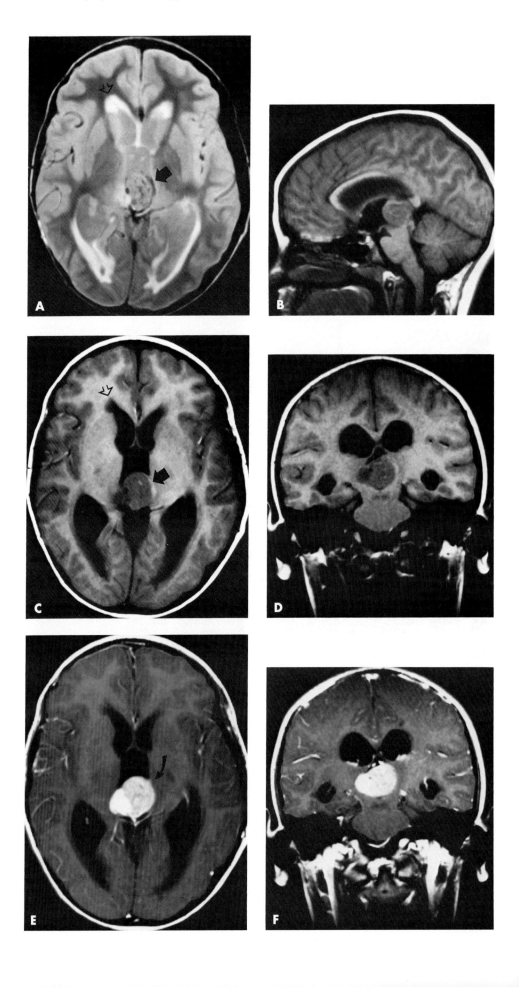

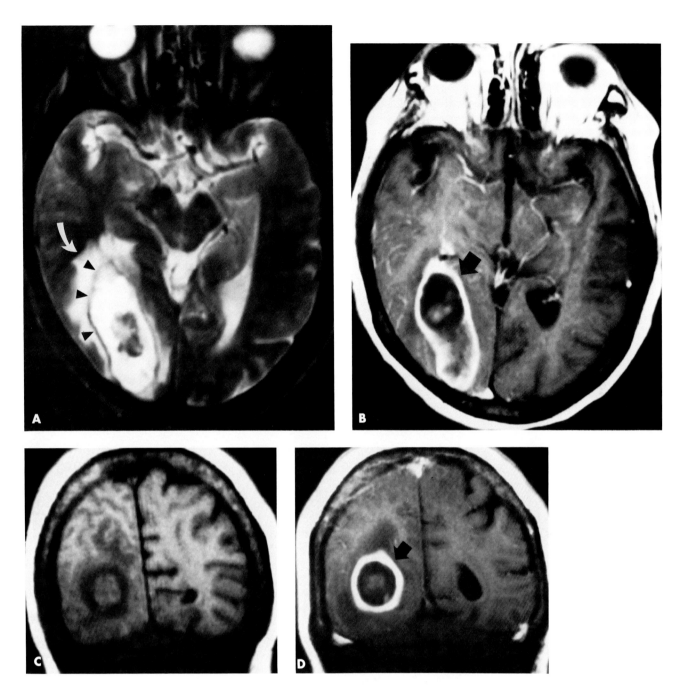

FIGURE 2-28. Right occipital brain abscess. **(A)** Axial T2-weighted, **(B)** postcontrast (gadopentetate dimeglumine) axial T1-weighted, and **(C, D)** precontrast and postcontrast coronal T1-weighted images. A 2 × 6-cm ring-enhancing lesion is noted in the right parieto-occipital region. The enhancing rim (*arrows*, **B, D**) is thick and uniform, suggesting the diagnosis of an abscess. The abscess capsule (*arrowheads*, **A**) can be faintly identified on the T2-weighted image as a low-signal intensity line separating central necrotic debris of high-signal intensity from surrounding high-signal intensity cerebral edema. There is considerable surrounding edema (*curved arrow*, **A**), with mass effect displacing the atria of the right lateral ventricle. This 65-year-old white woman presented with altered mental status and visual field cut. Frank pus (gram-postiive cocci) was identified at surgery, with drainage of the cavity and removal of the gliotic wall.

◄ **FIGURE 2-27.** Mixed germ cell tumor with dysgerminoma (seminoma) and immature teratoma elements. **(A)** Axial intermediate T2-weighted; **(B, C, D)** precontrast sagittal, axial, coronal T1-weighted; and **(E, F)** postcontrast (gadopentetate dimeglumine) axial and coronal T1-weighted images. This pineal tumor (*closed arrows*, **A, C**) is isointense precontrast relative to gray matter on both T1- and T2-weighted sequences. It has caused obstruction of the cerebral aqueduct with resultant hydrocephalus and transependymal flow (*open arrows*, **A, C**) noted on both T1- and T2-weighted images. There is uniform intense enhancement of the lesion postcontrast (*curved arrow*, **E**). The tumor was surgically excised with placement of a ventricular drain. This 9-year-old boy presented with several weeks of increasing headaches, nausea, and vomiting. Papilledema was noted on ophthalmic examination.

Infarction

The emphasis of early clinical trials with gadopentetate dimeglumine lay on the improved detection of neoplastic disease. Experience with paramagnetic metal ion chelates in cerebral infarction has been limited, with the value of contrast-enhanced scans largely unrecognized. In acute stroke, hypervascularity can be noted in the involved region (Fig. 2–34). If imaging is performed in the early hours following ictus, before the development of vasogenic edema, identification of hypervascularity can be the only sign of an acute stroke. Perfusion studies with rapid-imaging techniques such as turbo-FLASH can also be used during this time frame for improved lesion detection.

In the subacute period, there may be partial or near-total resolution of edema, as depicted by MRI, leading to difficulty in diagnosis on unenhanced scans. However, during this period, gyriform enhancement[42] occurs owing to disruption of the blood–brain barrier, making possible specific diagnosis on contrast-enhanced scans (Fig. 2–35). Japanese studies have documented the time course of lesion enhancement, with a gradual increase noted during the first hour after contrast injection.[43,44] Cortical and subcortical lesions, in particular, may be difficult to diagnose, with enhancement providing improved sensitivity. In addition to aiding lesion recognition, contrast administration can be of value by identifying gyriform enhancement (Fig. 2–36) and, thereby, improving the radiologist's ability to give a specific pathologic diagnosis (i.e., infarction).

A study of 50 patients presenting for MRI within 2 weeks of cerebellar infarction identified abnormal enhancement in 92%, with four phases of enhancing abnormalities identified.[45] The earliest finding, occurring in 17 of 22 infarcts 1 to 3 days of age, was enhancement of vessels within the anatomic area of involvement. From days 2 to 6, abnormal meningeal enhancement adjacent to the cortical infarct was frequently noted. From days 3 to 6, a transitional phase was seen, with early parenchymal enhancement combined with vascular or meningeal enhancement. The abnormal vascular enhancement noted in this series was attributed to engorgement and sluggish flow. Classic parenchymal enhancement was noted in all patients (17 of 17) imaged by MRI at 7 to 14 days after ictus.

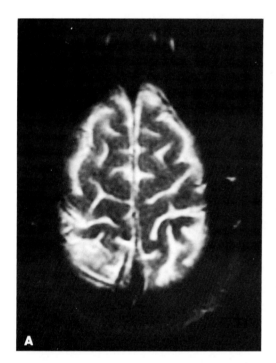
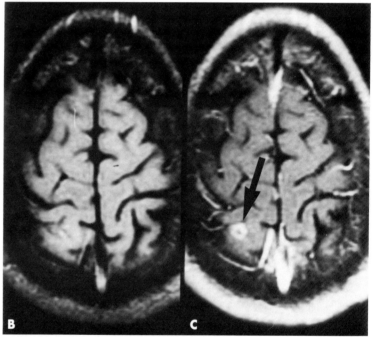

FIGURE 2–29. Toxoplasmosis in a 30-year-old man with AIDS who presented with left hemiparesis, numbness, and tingling. Precontrast axial T2-weighted **(A)** and T1-weighted **(B)** images; **(C)** axial postgadoteridol T1-weighted image. A right-sided ring-enhancing lesion (*arrow*, **C**) is best identified postcontrast. (Reprinted with permission from Runge VM, et al. Clinical safety and efficacy of gadoteridol (Gd HP-DO3A)—a study of 411 patients with suspected intracranial and spinal pathology. Radiology 1991;in press.)

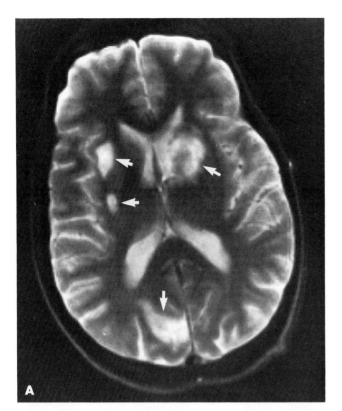

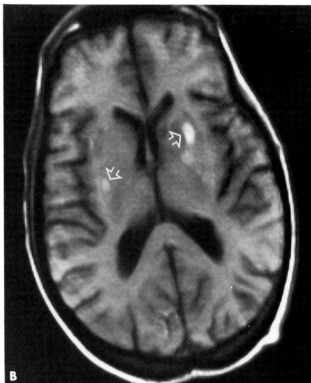

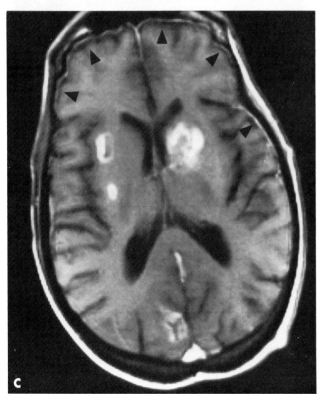

FIGURE 2-30. Acquired immunodeficiency syndrome (AIDS). Axial **(A)** T2-weighted and **(B, C)** precontrast and postcontrast T1-weighted images. Multiple high-signal intensity lesions can be noted on the precontrast T2-weighted examination (*white arrows*, **A**). Hemorrhage (methemoglobin, seen as high-signal intensity) is noted within several of these lesions (*open arrows*, **B**) on the precontrast T1-weighted examination. There is enhancement of each, following gadopentetate dimeglumine administration. Given the patient's history and clinical course, these findings were consistent with toxoplasmosis infection. On MRI, contrast enhancement can be used to assess disease activity in infection and differentiate an abscess capsule from surrounding edema. In this patient, there is also prominent enhancement of the dura (*arrowheads*, **C**), indicative of chronic meningeal disease. (Reprinted with permission from Runge VM, Gelblum DY. The role of gadolinium diethylene-triaminepentaacetic acid in the evaluation of the central nervous system. Magn Reson Q 1990;6:85–107)

In the elderly and hypertensive population, ischemic and gliotic changes can make the diagnosis of cerebral infarction difficult (Fig. 2–37). Contrast enhancement in this population has been efficacious for identification of lesions with blood–brain barrier disruption.[46]

Arteriovenous Abnormalities

Contrast administration can, by both direct and indirect means, improve the detection of arteriovenous abnormalities. In the last few years, motion compensation techniques have been implemented to improve the quality of routine head MR examinations. Unfortunately, this has decreased the sensitivity of MRI to vascular abnormalities, by changing the depiction of blood flow from that of a void to either iso- or hyperintensity. Contrast enhancement with gadolinium chelates, however, leads to a marked increase in signal intensity within blood vessels, a finding most prominent with slow flow in the venous system. Venous angiomas, in

particular, are thus best identified on postcontrast scans (Fig. 2–38). Contrast enhancement can also indirectly improve the identification of arteriovenous malformations (AVMs) and aneurysms. Pulsation artifacts from flowing blood are more prominent postcontrast, calling attention to the primary lesion itself. Unfortunately, contrast enhancement accentuates vascular pulsation artifacts from normal vessels, which can lead to overall image degradation on enhanced scans.[47] The use of gradient moment nulling can, in part, compensate for this effect, reducing vascular pulsation artifacts, and is recommended, in particular, on postcontrast scans. In MR angiography, administration of intravenous contrast provides improved portrayal of venous structures and small arteries.[48] When image reconstruction is performed using maximum-intensity projection techniques, lesions that enhance postcontrast are also seen on the projection images, an additional possible advantage. Vascular detail, however, can be obscured by enhance-

(Text continues on page 58)

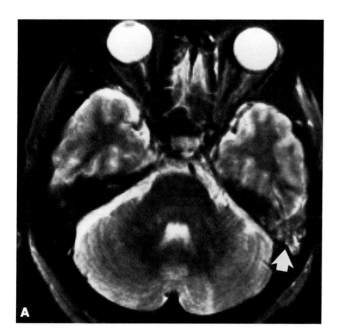
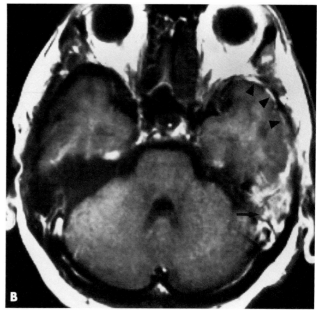

FIGURE 2–31. Mastoiditis with secondary meningitis in a 51-year-old man. Axial **(A)** precontrast T2-weighted and **(B)** postcontrast (gadopentetate dimeglumine) T1-weighted examinations. There is abnormal soft tissue, isointense with brain, identified on the precontrast T2-weighted examination in the left mastoid region (*white arrow,* **A**). Enhancement of the mass (*black arrow,* **B**) and meninges surrounding the left temporal lobe (*black arrowheads,* **B**) is noted postcontrast. Enhancement here permits the diagnosis of active infection. Infection in the frontal, mastoid, and petrous air cells can be difficult to diagnosis without contrast enhancement on MRI. Extension of enhancement outside the confines of the normal, air-filled sinus permits differentiation from more benign (and common) simple inflammation. (Reprinted with permission from Runge VM, Gelblum DY. The role of gadolinium diethylenetriaminepentaacetic acid in the evaluation of the central nervous system. Magn Reson Q 1990;6:85–107)

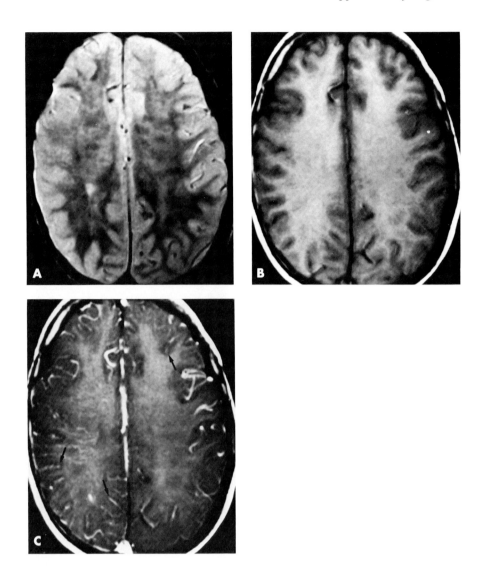

FIGURE 2–32. Postsurgical meningeal inflammation. Axial **(A)** T2-weighted and **(B, C)** precontrast and postcontrast (gadopentetate dimeglumine) T1-weighted images. There is diffuse enhancement of the pia–arachnoid (*arrows,* **C**). Disease involving the linings of the brain is often unidentified on unenhanced MRI, unless sufficiently large to be visualized as a mass lesion. This 13-year-old boy with neurofibromatosis presented with symptoms of cerebral ischemia, presumably secondary to radiation arteritis. The past medical history was significant for resection of a posterior fossa, low-grade astrocytoma.

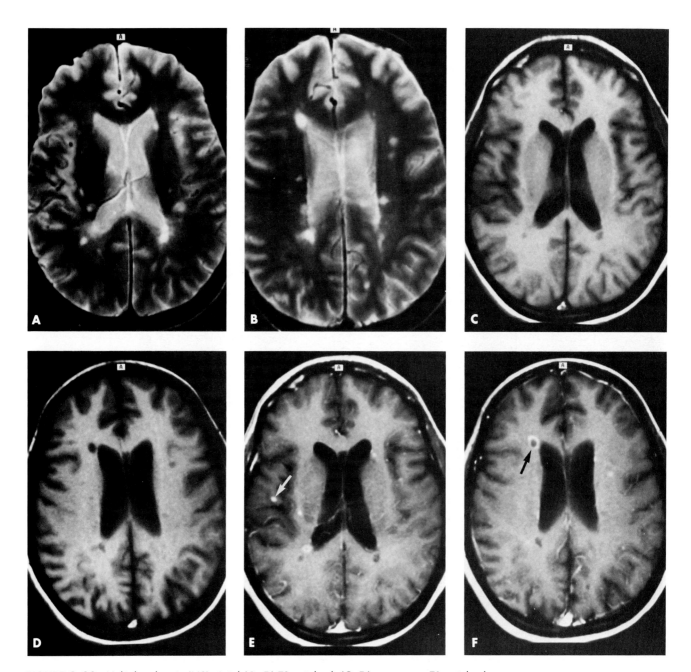

FIGURE 2–33. Multiple sclerosis (MS). Axial **(A, B)** T2-weighted, **(C, D)** precontrast T1-weighted, and **(E, F)** postcontrast (gadopentetate dimeglumine) T1-weighted images. On the T2-weighted examination multiple, punctate, periventricular, white matter, high-signal intensity abnormalities are noted. A few of these lesions demonstrate enhancement, both solid and ringlike (*black arrow,* **F**) in nature. Enhancement also permits identification of a more peripheral lesion (*white arrow,* **E**) adjacent to the right sylvian fissure. In MS, active lesions will demonstrate enhancement, with temporal progression from homogeneous to ringlike in nature. This 50-year-old white man had been diagnosed with multiple sclerosis for 14 years on the basis of right optic neuritis and spinal cord involvement. He is presently confined to a wheelchair with good upper-extremity strength. The patient presented for the current examination with increased incoordination in the upper extremities.

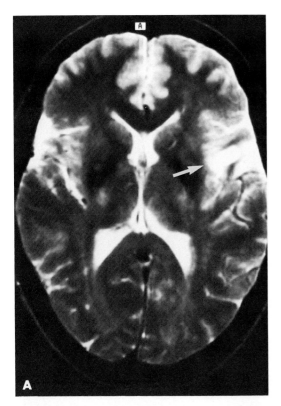

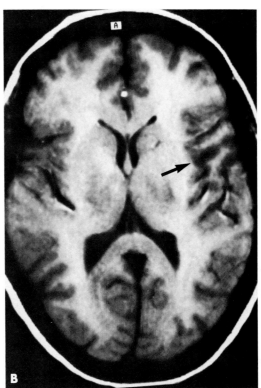

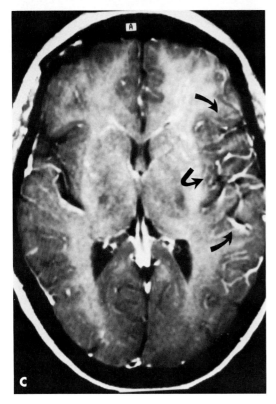

FIGURE 2–34. Acute left middle cerebral artery (MCA) infarction. Axial **(A)** T2-weighted and **(B, C)** precontrast and postcontrast (gadopentetate dimeglumine) T1-weighted examinations. There is abnormal high-signal intensity in the gray matter adjacent to the left sylvian fissure noted on the T2-weighted examination (*white arrow*, **A**). This is confirmed by the presence of abnormal low-signal intensity in the gray matter on the T1-weighted examination (*black arrow*, **B**). On the postcontrast examination, hypervascularity is noted in the MCA distribution (*curved arrows*, **C**). Increased vascular prominence ("luxury perfusion") can be the only abnormal finding in acute infarction on contrast-enhanced MRI, with disruption of the blood–brain barrier not commonly identified during this time frame. This 46-year-old woman presented with sudden onset of slurred speech 24 hours before the MR examination.

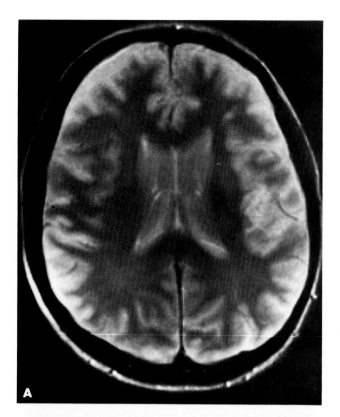

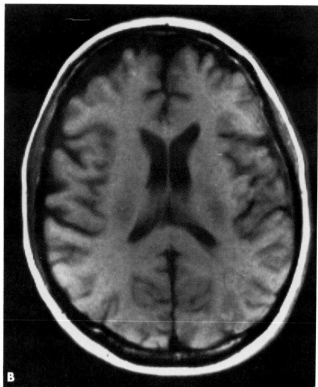

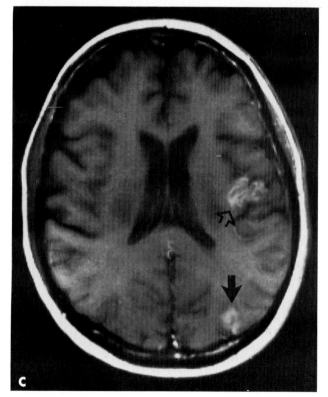

FIGURE 2–35. Subacute infarction. Axial **(A)** T2-weighted and **(B, C)** precontrast and postcontrast (gadopentetate dimeglumine) T1-weighted examinations. Slight hyperintensity on the T2-weighted examination in the left MCA distribution raises the question of cerebral infarction. Gyriform enhancement is identified on the postcontrast examination, both in the MCA distribution (*open arrow*, **C**) and in a watershed region (*black arrow*, **C**) between the MCA and PCA territories. As demonstrated by this case, in the subacute period, there may not be sufficient cerebral edema to identify infarction on unenhanced examinations. Disruption of the blood–brain barrier, with resultant gyriform enhancement permits definitive diagnosis. (Reprinted with permission from Runge VM, Gelblum DY. The role of gadolinium diethylenetriaminepentaacetic acid in the evaluation of the central nervous system. Magn Reson Q 1990;6:85–107)

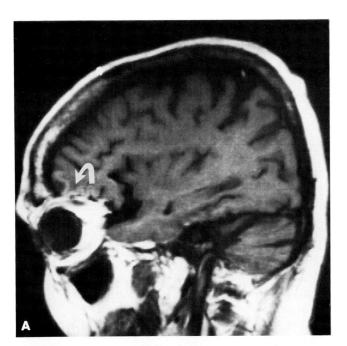

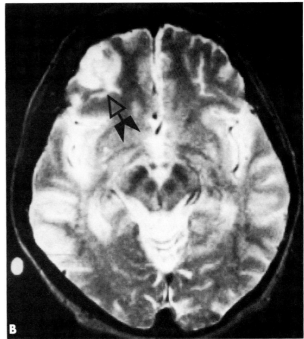

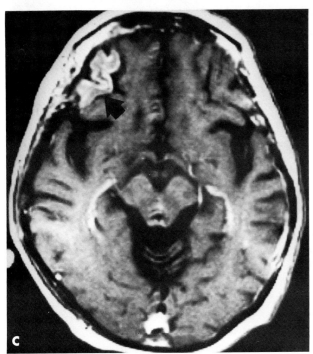

FIGURE 2-36. Infarction involving the orbital gyrus (anterior division, right middle cerebral artery) in a 62-year-old woman 45 days after acute presentation with loss of consciousness and dysarthria. Precontrast **(A)** sagittal T1-weighted and **(B)** axial T2-weighted images; **(C)** axial postgadoteridol T1-weighted image. There is gyriform enhancement postcontrast (*black arrow,* **C**), which improves lesion recognition and establishes the diagnosis of infarction. Vasogenic edema causes increased signal intensity on the T2-weighted scan (*open arrow,* **B**), although, on the heavily T2-weighted study, this is difficult to differentiate from chronic ischemic changes and cerebral atrophy. Petechial hemorrhage (*curved arrow,* **A**) lines the cortical surface of the involved region on the sagittal precontrast T1-weighted image. (Reprinted with permission from Runge, VM, et al. Phase III clinical evaluation of Gd HP-DO3A in head and spine disease. Magn Reson Imaging 1991;1:47–56)

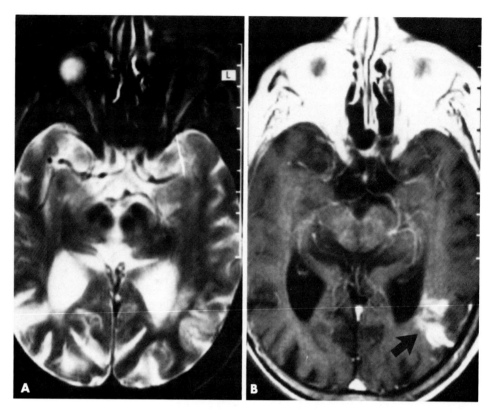

FIGURE 2–37. Subacute watershed infarction in a 74-year-old woman. The patient presented with expressive aphasia 3½-weeks before MR examination. Axial **(A)** precontrast T2-weighted and **(B)** post gadoteridol T1-weighted images. The lesion was only slightly hyperintense relative to normal brain on both echoes of the precontrast T2-weighted examination. Because of extensive chronic ischemic and gliotic white matter changes, identification of this lesion prospectively on unenhanced scans was difficult. Demarcation of blood–brain barrier disruption (*black arrow,* **B**) following administration of gadoteridol was felt to improve lesion visualization, lesion detection, and disease classification in this patient (who was part of a Phase III clinical trial). (Reprinted with permission from Runge VM, et al. Clinical safety and efficacy of gadoteridol (Gd HP-DO3A)—a study of 411 patients with suspected intracranial and spinal pathology. Radiology 1991;in press)

ment of extracranial tissues, in particular the nasal mucosa; hence, MR angiography is typically performed before the administration of intravenous contrast.

CONTRAST MEDIA IN CLINICAL PRACTICE

New Agents

Several new agents have been evaluated for improved head imaging in recent clinical trials. All fall within the class of paramagnetic metal ion chelates and employ the gadolinium ion for relaxation effects. In the United States, both gadoteridol (Gd-HP-DO3A; ProHance, Squibb Diagnostics, Princeton, New Jersey)[49,50] and gadodiamide (Gd-DTPA-BMA; Omniscan, Winthrop Pharmaceuticals, New York, New York)[51] have completed Phase III investigation and have been submitted for FDA approval. Both of these new agents are non-

ionic. Phase II and III investigations with gadoteridol have been pursued with doses up to 0.3 mmol/kg, three times that approved for gadopentetate dimeglumine. Preliminary results suggest greater efficacy at higher administered dose, particularly with intracranial metastatic disease. The approval of gadoteridol for routine clinical use is anticipated within the next year. Its availability is likely to significantly change clinical practice, with high-dose contrast studies thus feasible.

Gadoterate meglumine (Gd-DOTA; Dotarem, Guerbet, France)[52,53] although not introduced in the United States, was developed after gadopentetate dimeglumine, and is approved for clinical use in several European and South American nations. Compared with Gd-DTPA, which has a –2 charge, gadoterate has a –1 charge and, hence, requires only a single positive ion for preparation as a water-soluble ionic compound. Recent work has also been published from Schering AG with gadopentetate dimeglumine-bismorpholide,[54] a lower-osmolality agent.

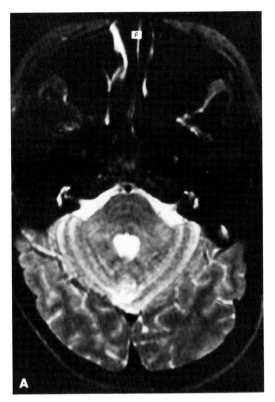

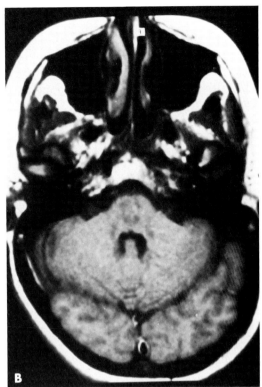

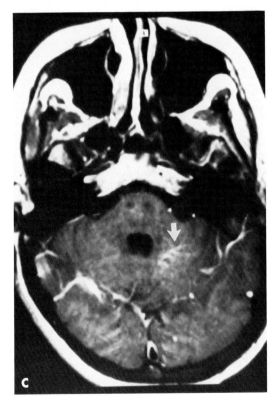

FIGURE 2–38. Left superior cerebellar venous angioma. Axial **(A)** T2-weighted and **(B, C)** precontrast and postcontrast (gadopentetate dimeglumine) T1-weighted images. The use of motion-compensating software techniques, such as gradient moment refocusing (GMR), on both T1- and T2-weighted examinations on state-of-the-art clinical MR systems has resulted in a loss of sensitivity to small vascular lesions. Enhancement of slow blood flow within this venous anomaly permits not only recognition of the lesion (*arrow*, **C**), but definitive diagnosis, by identification of the "caput" of draining veins. Arterial and venous enhancement can be observed on MRI after IV administration of a paramagnetic metal ion chelate, with resultant improved diagnosis of arteriovenous malformations.

With all gadolinium chelates, emphasis has been placed on achieving high stability of the complex in vivo, preventing release of the free metal ion and, thereby, potentially lowering toxicity. Gadoteridol and gadoterate meglumine exhibit remarkable stability here, resisting transmetalation with zinc or copper ions far better than gadopentetate dimeglumine.

The only blood abnormality noted following gadopentetate dimeglumine administration has been a transient rise in serum iron and bilirubin levels.[55] It has been hypothesized that this transient change is due to blood hemolysis. No consistent laboratory changes have been noted to be caused by gadoteridol administration in clinical trials.

Contrast Dose

There was little experience in 1983 to guide the initial choice of 0.1 mmol/kg as the standard dose for gadopentetate dimeglumine. Phase I trials covered a broad range of dosages and revealed consistent drug-related hematologic abnormalities of unclear etiology (at that time) at higher doses. These results favored the choice of a dose of 0.1 mmol/kg, or less, yet most animal investigations had been conducted with 0.25 mmol/kg. Fortunately, initial Phase II clinical investigations subsequently performed in Germany that used a dose of 0.1 mmol/kg revealed excellent lesion enhancement.

In the years since 1983, only limited clinical studies examining the question of dosage have been performed. Investigation with gadopentetate dimeglumine focused primarily on lower doses, which were shown not to be efficacious (Fig. 2–39), although limited results at higher doses (0.2 mmol/kg) suggested increased "diagnostic yield."[56]

Phase II studies with gadoteridol in 1989 marked the first time in the United States in which doses larger than 0.1 mmol/kg of a gadolinium chelate were examined for lesion enhancement. Gadolinium chelates produce lesion enhancement by facilitating T1 relaxation. However, these agents similarly facilitate T2 relaxation. The two effects are competing, with a reduction in T1 causing an increase in signal intensity and a reduction in T2 causing a decrease in signal intensity on spin echo imaging. Thus, the question of optimum dose for a paramagnetic contrast agent becomes much more complex than with iodinated agents and x-ray–based modalities, since too high concentrations of a gadolinium chelate can actually result in *negative* enhancement. The latter situation can actually be observed in routine lumbar spine imaging (at 0.1 mmol/kg), with the bladder and renal collecting systems becoming markedly hypointense (as opposed to hyperintense as with x-ray agents) postcontrast owing to hyper-

concentration of the agent. Despite the potential for decreased or less efficacious enhancement at high administered dose, both theoretical studies and animal experimentation favored greater lesion enhancement at doses up to 0.3 mmol/kg (and perhaps higher) in brain studies. This was confirmed in the previously described Phase II clinical trials for gadoteridol, with both doses of 0.2 and 0.3 mmol/kg resulting in a substantial improvement in lesion enhancement, compared with a 0.1-mmol/kg dose (Fig. 2–40).

Phase III high-dose trials with gadoteridol are now in progress and are designed specifically to investigate efficacy in the examination of intracranial metastatic disease. In preliminary results from 12 patients,[57] lesion enhancement more than doubled when comparing a dose of 0.1 mmol/kg with one of 0.3 mmol/kg (Fig. 2–41). In certain cases, lesions were detected prospectively only following high-dose contrast administration (Fig. 2–42). Additional observations included improved demonstration of enhancement in hemorrhagic metastases (Fig. 2–43)—in which enhancement can be difficult to detect at standard contrast dosage owing to the hyperintensity of the lesions precontrast—and the apparent increase in size of certain lesions as depicted on high-dose, compared with standard-dose, examinations. Limited experience with disorders other than metastatic disease suggests that improved lesion enhancement is likely regardless of disease etiology at high-contrast dose on MRI (Fig. 2–44). No adverse effects related to high-dose contrast administration have yet been observed in these limited trials.

Clinical Use

Three prospective studies[58–60] have evaluated the efficacy of contrast administration, specifically with gadopentetate dimeglumine, in MR examination of the head. In a study by Runge and co-workers, contrast administration significantly changed scan interpretation in 25% of all cases.[58] Both the failure to recognize a lesion (5%) and misdiagnosis (20%) occurred on interpretation of precontrast scans alone. In this limited study of 225 patients, lesions that went undiagnosed on precontrast studies included acoustic neuromas, subacute infarction, and vascular abnormalities. Overall, 68% of abnormal head examinations benefited in terms of additional diagnostic information from contrast administration. In the study by Elster and associates, lesions were apparent on contrast enhancement alone in 3% of cases.[59] In this series of 500 patients, contrast enhancement was viewed to be helpful in diagnosis in 15%, with the lack of enhancement benefiting an additional 22%. In the study by Schwaighofer and colleagues, 8 of the 514 patients had negative precontrast studies with one or more lesions identified only on

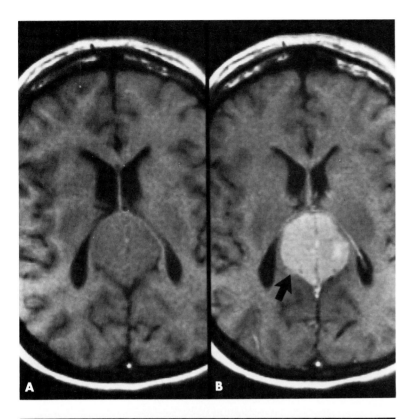

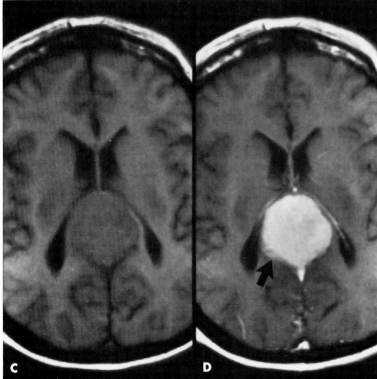

FIGURE 2-39. Tentorial meningioma, comparing enhancement with 0.05 (low-dose) and 0.1 mmol/kg (standard-dose). **(A, B)** Pre- and postcontrast (0.05-mmol/kg IV gadoteridol) T1-weighted images. **(C, D)** Pre- and postcontrast (0.1-mmol/kg IV gadopentetate dimeglumine) T1-weighted images. Lesion enhancement (*arrows,* **B, D**) is noted at both doses. However, enhancement is marginal at the low dose, despite the fact that the lesion illustrated is one that typically demonstrates intense enhancement. Quantitatively, the percentage lesion enhancement was 26% at 0.05 mmol/kg and 48% at 0.1 mmol/kg. Preliminary data do not support use of contrast doses less than 0.1 mmol/kg for visualization of brain lesions. (Reprinted with permission from Runge VM, et al. Gd HP-DO3A in clinical MR imaging of the brain. Radiology 1990;177:393–400)

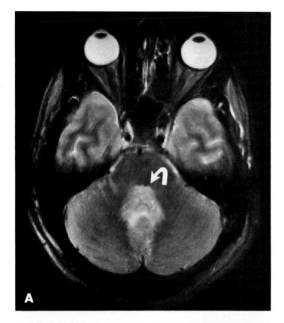

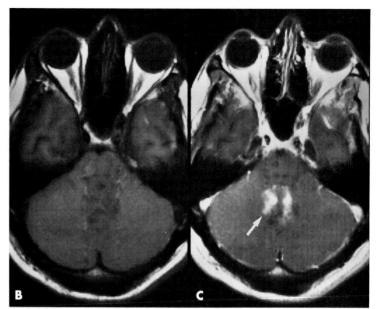

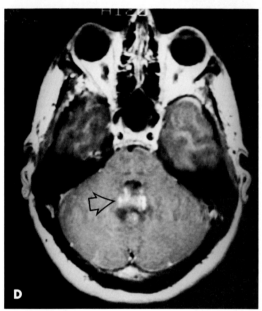

FIGURE 2–40. Desmoplastic medulloma, comparing enhancement with 0.1 (standard dose) and 0.3 mmol/kg (high dose). Axial **(A)** T2-weighted, **(B)** precontrast T1-weighted, **(C)** after 0.3 mmol/kg of gadoteridol, and **(D)** after 0.1 mmol/kg of gadopentetate dimeglumine. The lesion (*curved arrow,* **A**) is slightly hyperintense relative to adjacent brain on the T2-weighted image. Portions of the lesion (*white arrow,* **C**) demonstrate intense enhancement at a contrast dose of 0.3 mmol/kg. Abnormal contrast enhancement (*open arrow,* **D**) is less well visualized at the standard dose of 0.1 mmol/kg. (Reprinted with permission from Runge VM, et al. Gd HP-DO3A in clinical MR imaging of the brain. Radiology 1990;177:393–400)

postcontrast images.[60] In comparison with the other two studies, the number of contrast-enhancing lesions in this series of patients was significantly lower (11%).

In the few years since FDA approval (mid-1988), gadopentetate dimeglumine has been recognized as a valuable adjunct in head MR imaging. Concern for medical costs has no doubt restricted its use. Caution is advised, as with all IV agents, because of the possibility of an anaphylactic reaction. Such agents should be administered under a physician's supervision, with attention to proper training and availability of resuscitation equipment, in concert with the approach used for iodinated agents with radiographic-based imaging.

In many instances, including small extra-axial lesions, metastatic disease, subacute infarction, infection, and meningeal disease, detection of disease is possible on MRI only following contrast administration. Although such is not required for the identification of larger tumors, contrast administration in this instance does improve lesion definition and facilitates scan interpretation. In the postoperative patient, contrast enhancement is mandatory for identification of residual or recurrent tumor.

New agents like gadoteridol offer the potential for high-dose administration. Such agents may indeed prove safer, as suggested by in vitro results demon-

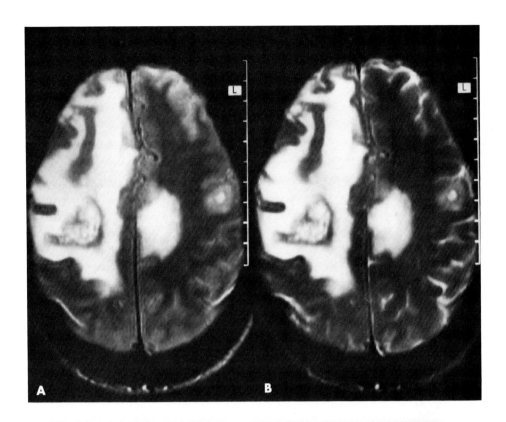

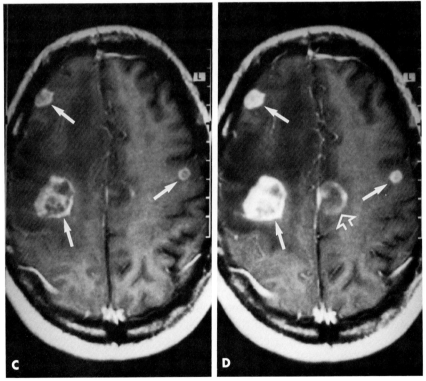

FIGURE 2-41. Metastatic lung carcinoma, demonstrating superior lesion enhancement at high-contrast dose (0.3 mmol/kg) with gadoteridol. **(A, B)** First and second echoes from the precontrast T2-weighted examination. Axial T1-weighted images **(C)** immediately after administration of 0.1 mmol/kg IV gadoteridol and **(D)** immediately after 0.3 mmol/kg (cumulative dose) IV gadoteridol. Several lesions can be identified on the precontrast T2-weighted examination, principally on the basis of the cerebral edema elicited. Definite enhancement of three lesions is noted (*arrows,* **C**) following a contrast dose of 0.1 mmol/kg. At the 0.3 mmol/kg dose, the enhancement of each of these lesions (*arrows,* **D**) improves markedly, with additional demonstration of ring enhancement of a parafalcine lesion (*open arrow,* **D**). In retrospect, this fourth lesion demonstrates faint enhancement at the 0.1-mmol/kg dose. (Reprinted with permission from Runge VM, et al. High dose application of gadoteridol in brain MRI. In press)

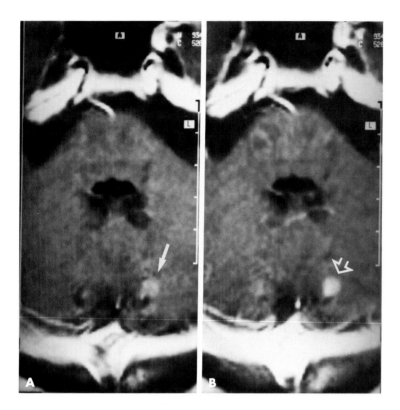

FIGURE 2–42. Metastatic lung carcinoma, demonstrating nonvisualization of a neoplastic lesion after a 0.1-mmol/kg IV contrast dose, with lesion detection permitted only because of subsequent utilization of high-dose gadoteridol injection. Axial T1-weighted images immediately after **(A)** 0.1 mmol/kg and **(B)** 0.3 mmol/kg (cumulative dose) gadoteridol. The lesion was not detected on T2-weighted images (not illustrated) prospectively by two readers blinded to clinical history. Each reader also failed to detect this cerebellar metastasis on the 0.1-mmol/kg postcontrast examination, with identification of the lesion made in each case only on the 0.3-mmol/kg postcontrast examination. This lesion was confirmed by repeat examination with thin-section imaging. The faint enhancement at the 0.1-mmol/kg dose (*arrow*, **A**) is not sufficient to permit lesion detection, which was made without difficulty after high-dose contrast administration (*open arrow*, **B**). (Reprinted with permission from Runge VM, et al. High dose application of gadoteridol in brain MRI. In press)

strating greater stability relative to metal ion exchange, clearance studies from animal experimentation, and human trials[61] (which to date reveal no clinically significant change in laboratory parameters). High-dose contrast administration should have an immediate impact in the study of metastatic disease, with more widespread clinical efficacy likely.

The use of contrast enhancement in MRI is still guided largely by the index of clinical suspicion. Recent work[62] recommends routine use in head examinations, excluding only two categories, that of young adults and of children with normal unenhanced studies. Guidelines for pediatric use have also evolved from clinical trials.[63] Little data exists regarding contrast administration in neonates, in whom glomerular filtration and, consequently, renal clearance are significantly reduced. Preliminary safety and efficacy data were obtained in a recent study of 15 neonates and young infants.[64] Four of 15 patients had significant abnormalities on the postcontrast scan that were not demonstrated precontrast. Vivid contrast enhancement of normal structures, which persisted for several hours following injection, presumably on the basis of reduced clearance rates, was demonstrated in this population.

Gadopentetate dimeglumine is the first agent to receive FDA approval, combining high efficacy with a high degree of safety.[65] Clinical indications for contrast administration are extensive, with widespread clinical use.[66–68] Approval of second-generation agents, such as gadoteridol, will likely lead to a further major advance in diagnostic use.

REFERENCES

1. Weinmann HJ, Brasch RC, Press WR, Wesbey GE. Characterization of gadolinium-DTPA complex: a potential NMR contrast agent. AJR 1984;142:619.

2. Runge VM, Stewart RG, Clanton JA, et al. Paramagnetic NMR contrast agents: potential oral and intravenous agents. Radiology 1983;147:789.

3. Felix R, Schorner W, Laniado M, et al. Brain tumors: MR imaging with gadolinium-DTPA. Radiology 1985;156:681.

4. Carr DH, Brown J, Bydder GM, et al. Gadolinium DTPA as a contrast agent in MRI: initial clinical experience in 20 patients. AJR 1984;143:215.

5. Brant-Zawadzki M, Berry I, Osaki L, et al. Gadolinium DTPA in clinical MR of the brain. I. Intra-axial lesions. AJNR 1986;7:781.

6. Runge VM, Schaible TF, Goldstein HA, et al. Gadopentetate dimeglumine—clinical efficacy. Radiographics 1988;8:147–159.

7. Runge VM, ed. Enhanced magnetic resonance imaging. St Louis: CV Mosby, 1989.

8. Schmiedl U, Maravilla KR, Gerlach R, et al. Excretion of gadopentetate dimeglumine in human breast milk. AJR 1990;154:1305–1306.

9. Runge VM, Gelblum DY, Wood ML. 3-D imaging of the CNS. Neuroradiology 1990;32:356–366.

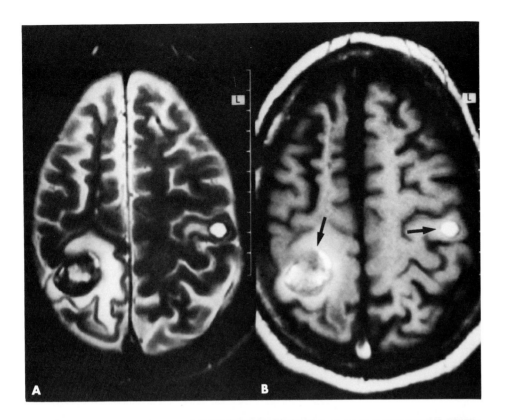

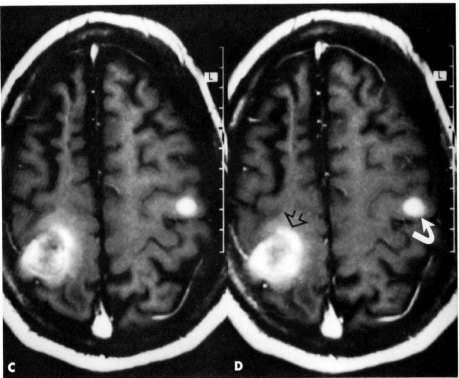

FIGURE 2–43. Metastatic lung carcinoma, demonstrating improved detection of lesion enhancement at high-contrast dose with gadoteridol in the presence of intracranial hemorrhage. Precontrast axial **(A)** T2-weighted and **(B)** T1-weighted images. Axial postcontrast T1-weighted images immediately after gadoteridol injection with a dose of **(C)** 0.1 mmol/kg and **(D)** 0.3 mmol/kg (cumulative). Two hemorrhagic lesions are seen precontrast (*black arrows,* **B**). There is subtle contrast enhancement of the larger right-sided lesion at the 0.1-mmol/kg dose, which is demonstrated with confidence at high dose (*open black arrow,* **D**). The indistinctness of the margins of the smaller left-sided metastasis (*curved white arrow,* **D**) on the high-dose examination is also due to subtle enhancement. (Reprinted with permission from Runge, VM, et al. High dose application of gadoteridol in brain MRI. In press)

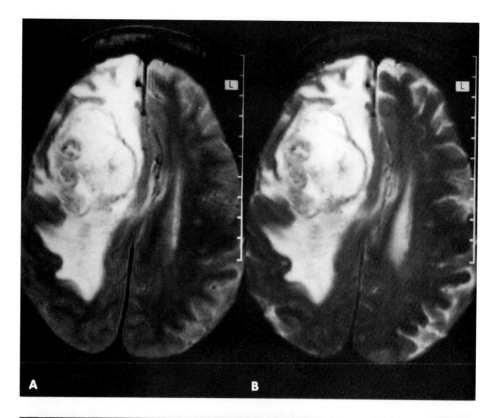

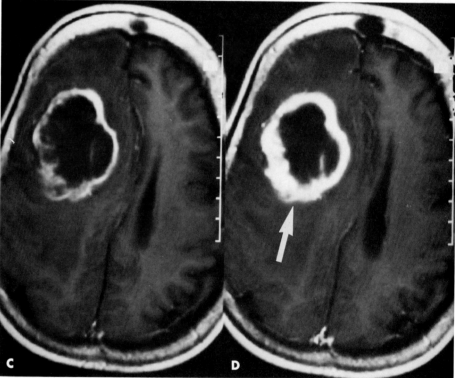

FIGURE 2–44. Glioblastoma multiforme, demonstrating improved depiction of blood–brain barrier disruption (by greater enhancement) at high-contrast dose with gadoteridol. **(A, B)** First and second echoes from the precontrast T2-weighted examination, axial T1-weighted images **(C)** immediately after 0.1 mmol/kg IV gadoteridol and **(D)** immediately after 0.3 mmol/kg (cumulative dose) IV gadoteridol. The rim of contrast enhancement is thicker and more prominent at high-dose (*arrow,* **D**). Statistically, a 116% improvement was noted in lesion enhancement at the 0.3-mmol/kg, compared with the 0.1-mmol/kg contrast dose. (Reprinted with permission from Runge VM, et al. High dose application of gadoteridol in brain MRI. In press)

10. Weiss KL. Severe anaphylactoid reaction after IV Gd-DTPA. Magn Reson Imaging 1990;8:817–818.

11. Haughton VM, Rimm AA, Czervionke LF, et al. Sensitivity of Gd-DTPA enhanced MR imaging of benign extra-axial tumors. Radiology 1988;166:829–833.

12. Nelson KL, Runge VM. Radiologic evaluation of acoustic neuromas. Magn Reson Imaging Decis 1987;1:31.

13. Stack JP, Ramsden RT, Antoun NM, et al. Magnetic resonance imaging of acoustic neuromas: the role of gadolinium DTPA. Br J Radiol 1988;61:800–805.

14. Litt AW, Kindo N, Bannon KR, Kricheff II. Role of slice thickness in MR imaging of the internal auditory canal. J Comput Assist Tomogr 1990;14:717–720.

15. Cass SP, Kartush JM, Wilner HI, Graham MD. Comparison of computerized tomography and magnetic resonance imaging for the postoperative assessment of residual acoustic tumor. Otolaryngol Head Nect Surg 1991;104:182–190.

16. Bydder GM, Kingsley DPE, Brown J, et al. MR imaging of meningioma including studies with and without gadolinium DTPA. J Comput Assist Tomogr 1985;9:690.

17. Claussen C, Laniado M, Schorner W, et al. Gadolinium DTPA in imaging of glioblastomas and intracranial metastases. AJNR 1985;6:669.

18. Powers TA, Partain CL, Kessler RM, et al. Central nervous system lesions in pediatric patients: Gd-DTPA-enhanced MR imaging. Radiology 1988;169:723–726.

19. Forsting M, Albert FK, Sartor K. Baseline CT and MRI after brain resection: prognostic value [abstract]. American Society of Neuroradiology annual meeting, June 1991:29.

20. Healy ME, Hesselink JR, Press GA, Middleton MS. Increased detection of intracranial metastases with intravenous gadopentetate dimeglumine. Radiology 1987;165:619.

21. Bird CR, Drayer BP, Medina M, et al. Gadopentetate dimeglumine-enhanced MR imaging in pediatric patients after brain tumor resection. Radiology 1988;169:123–126.

22. Rollins N, Mendelsohn D, Mulne A, et al. Recurrent medulloblastoma: frequency of tumor enhancement on Gd-DTPA MR imaging. AJNR 1990;11:583–587.

23. Grossman RI, Hecht-Leavitt CM, Evans SM, et al. Experimental radiation injury: combined MR imaging and spectroscopy. Radiology 1988;169:305–309.

24. West MS, Russell EJ, Breit R, et al. Calvarial and skull base metastases: comparison of nonenhanced and gadopentetate dimeglumine-enhanced MR images. Radiology 1990;174:85.

25. Doppman JL, Frank JA, Dwyer AJ, et al. Gadolinium DTPA enhanced MR imaging of ACTH-secreting microadenomas of the pituitary gland. J Comput Assist Tomogr 1988;12:728–735.

26. Wichmann W, Schubiger O, Valavanis A, Kasdaglis K. MR diagnosis of microadenomas of the pituitary gland. ROFO 1988;149:239–244.

27. Newton DR, Dillon WP, Norman D, et al. Gd-DTPA-enhanced MR imaging of pituitary adenomas. AJNR 1989;10:949–954.

28. Runge VM, Clanton JA, Price AC, et al. Evaluation of contrast-enhanced MR imaging in a brain abscess model. AJNR 1985;6:139–147.

29. Mathews VP, Kuharik MA, Edwards MK, et al. Gd-DTPA-enhanced MR imaging of experimental bacterial meningitis: evaluation and comparison with CT. AJNR 1988;9:1045–1050.

30. Chang KH, Han MH, Roh JK, et al. Gd-DTPA enhanced MR imaging of the brain in patients with meningitis: comparison with CT. AJR 1990;154:809–816.

31. Frank JA, Girton M, Dwyer AJ, et al. Meningeal carcinomatosis in the VX2 rabbit tumor model: detection with Gd-DTPA enhanced MR imaging. Radiology 1988;167:825–829.

32. Elster AD, DiPersio DA. Cranial postoperative site: assessment with contrast-enhanced MR imaging. Radiology 1990;174:93–98.

33. Schorner W, Henkes H, Sander B, Felix R. MR demonstration of the meninges: normal and pathological findings. ROFO 1988;149:361–368.

34. Lee YY, Tien RD, Bruner JM, et al. Loculated intracranial leptomeningeal metastases: CT and MR characteristics. AJR 1990;154:351–359.

35. Burke JW, Podrasky AE, Bradley, WG. Jr. Meninges: benign postoperative enhancement of MR images. Radiology 1990;174:99–102.

36. Miller DH, Rudge P, Johnson G, et al. Serial gadolinium enhanced magnetic resonance imaging in multiple sclerosis. Brain 1988;111:927–939.

37. Grossman RI, Gonzalez-Scarano F, Atlas SW, et al. Multiple sclerosis: gadolinium enhancement in MR imaging. Radiology 1986;161:721.

38. Kermode AG, Thompson AJ, Tofts P, et al. Breakdown of the blood–brain barrier precedes symptoms and other MRI signs of new lesions in multiple sclerosis. Pathogenetic and clinical implications. Brain 1990;113:1477–1489.

39. Bastianello S, Pozzilli C, Bernardi S, et al. Serial study of gadolinium-DTPA MRI enhancement in multiple sclerosis. Neurology 1990;40:591–595.

40. Larsson HB, Stubgaard M, Frederiksen JL, et al. Quantitation of blood–brain barrier defect by magnetic resonance imaging and gadolinium-DTPA in patients with multiple sclerosis and brain tumors. Magn Reson Med 1990;16:117–131.

41. Larsson EM, Holtas S, Nilsson O. Gd-DTPA–enhanced MR of suspected spinal multiple sclerosis. AJNR 1989;10:1071–1076.

42. Virapongse C, Mancuso AA, Quisling RG. Human brain infarcts: imaging by MR enhanced gadopentetate dimeglumine. Radiology 1986;161:785.

43. Imakita S, Nishimura T, Yamada N, et al. Magnetic resonance imaging of cerebral infarction: time course of Gd-DTPA enhancement and CT comparison. Neuroradiology 1988;30:372–378.

44. Miyashita K, Naritomi H, Sawada T, et al. Identification of recent lacunar lesions in cases of multiple small infarctions by magnetic resonance imaging. Stroke 1988;19:834–839.

45. Elster AD, Moody DM. Early cerebral infarction: gadopentetate dimeglumine enhancement. Radiology 1990;177:627–632.

46. Runge VM. Contrast media. In: Runge VM, ed. Clinical magnetic resonance imaging. Philadelphia: JB Lippincott, 1990:535.

47. Richardson DN, Elster AD, et al. Gd-DTPA-enhanced MR images: accentuation of vascular pulsation artifacts and correction by using gradient-moment nulling (MAST). AJNR 1990;11:209–210.

48. Creasy JL, Price RR, Presbrey T, et al. Gadolinium-enhanced MR angiography. Radiology 1990;175:280–283.

49. Runge VM, Gelblum DY, Pacetti ML, et al. Gd HP-DO3A in clinical MR imaging of the brain. Radiology 1990;177:393–400.

50. Runge V, Dean B, Lee C, et al. Phase III clinical evaluation of Gd HP-DO3A in head and spine disease. J Magn Reson Imaging 1991;1:47–56.

51. Greco A, McNamara MT, Lanthiez P, et al. Gadodiamide injection: nonionic gadolinium chelate for MR imaging of the brain and spine—phase II–III clinical trial. Radiology 1990;176:451–456.

52. Meyer D, Schaefer M, Bonnemain B. Gd-DOTA, a potential MRI contrast agent: current status of physicochemical knowledge. Invest Radiol 1988;23(suppl 1):S232–235.

53. Allard M, Doucet D, Kien P, et al. Experimental study of DOTA-gadolinium: pharmacokinetics and pharmacologic properties. Invest Radiol 1988;23(suppl 1):S271–274.

54. Aicher KP, White DL, Dupon JW, et al. Gadopentetate dimeglumine-bismorpholide, a new low-osmolar contrast agent for MR imaging. Radiology 1989;173(suppl):365.

55. Niendorf HP, Seifert W. Serum iron and serum bilirubin after administration of Gd-DTPA-dimeglumine: a pharmacologic study in health volunteers. Invest Radiol 1988;23(suppl 1):S275–280.

56. Niendorf HP, Laniado M, Semmler W, et al. Dose administration of gadolinium DTPA in MR imaging of intracranial tumors. AJNR 1987;8:803–815.

57. Runge VM, Kirsch JE, Burke V, et al. High dose application of gadoteridol in brain MRI (in press).

58. Carollo BR, Runge VM, Price AC, et al. The prospective evaluation of Gd-DTPA in 225 consecutive cranial cases: adverse reactions and diagnostic value. Magn Reson Imaging 1990;8:381–393.

59. Elster AD, Moody DM, Ball MR, Laster DW. Is Gd-DTPA required for routine cranial MR imaging? Radiology 1989;173:231–238.

60. Schwaighofer BW, Klein MV, Wesbey G, Hesselink JR. Clinical experience with routine Gd-DTPA administration for MR imaging of the brain. J Comput Assist Tomogr 1990;14:11–17.

61. Runge VM, Bradley WG, Brant-Zawadzki MN, et al. Clinical safety and efficacy of gadoteridol (Gd HP-DO3A)—a study of 411 patients with suspected intracranial and spinal pathology. Radiology 1991; (in press).

62. Runge VM, Gelblum DY. The role of gadolinium-diethylene-triaminepentaacetic acid in the evaluation of the central nervous system. Magn Reson Q 1990;6:85–107.

63. Elster AD, Reister GD. Gd-DTPA enhanced cranial MR imaging in children: initial clinical experience and recommendations for its use. AJNR 1989;10:1027–1030.

64. Elster AD. Cranial MR imaging with Gd-DTPA in neonates and young infants: preliminary experience. Radiology 1990;176:225–230.

65. Goldstein HA, Kashanian FK, Blumetti RF, et al. Safety assessment of gadopentetate dimeglumine in U.S. clinical trials. Radiology 1990;174:17–23.

66. Runge VM, Carollo BR, Wolf CR, et al. Gadopentetate dimeglumine: a review of clinical indications in central nervous system magnetic resonance imaging. Radiographics 1989;9:929–958.

67. Bauer WM, Fenzl G, Vogl TH, et al. Indications for the use of Gd-DTPA in MRI of the central nervous system. Experiences in patients with cerebral and spinal disease. Invest Radiol 1988;23:S286–288.

68. Runge VM. Contrast media in magnetic resonance imaging. In: Clinical applications of magnetic resonance imaging 1989. Prepared by the American College of Radiology Committee on Clinical Applications, p. 60.

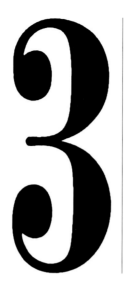

Clinical Applications of Magnetic Resonance Contrast Media in the Spine

Bruce L. Dean
Charles Lee

IMAGING STRATEGIES

An optimal magnetic resonance (MR)-imaging strategy of the spine should be based on the region of anatomic interest and the type of lesion suspected. Manipulation of the pulse sequences can highlight structures of interest and, when coupled with intravenous injection of a paramagnetic contrast agent, can enhance normal anatomy as well as functional or structural abnormalities.

Depending on the pulse sequence selected, optimal imaging of the vertebral body and its posterior elements, intervertebral disk, neuroforamina, spinal cord, cerebrospinal fluid (CSF), and vascular structures can be achieved. Choice of imaging techniques on most commercial MR imagers includes T1- and T2-weighted spin echo pulse sequences, and gradient echo imaging including FISP, FLASH, and GRASS sequences. The MR contrast agents, at currently accepted clinical doses, exhibit shortening predominantly of the T1 relaxation time. Therefore, T1-weighted pulse sequences are mandatory to maximize the contrast-enhancing properties. Motion and fat suppression techniques are also useful. Other MR techniques that have not been fully developed include CSF flow imaging, fat/water chemical shift imaging, and spectroscopy.

T1-Weighted Spin Echo Imaging of the Normal Spine

For maximal spatial resolution T1-weighted spin echo pulse sequences are the method of choice, highlighting the vertebral bodies and their posterior elements, spinal cord, intervertebral disks, and vertebral venous structures as intermediate-signal intensity or gray structures. Epidural fat and CSF appear as white and black, respectively, an appearance that further delineates the

dural sac and spinal cord by the contrast differences at the cord–CSF interface (Fig. 3–1). The epidural fat–nerve root interface allows excellent visualization of the neuroforamen and its exiting nerve root sleeve on the sagittal images (see Fig. 3–1). Because high-resolution detail is important, a 256 × 256 matrix is used. Both axial and sagittal views are obtained.

The axial view is important for assessing canal and lateral recess size, as well as for lateralization of herniated disk or spurs. The sagittal view is also important for localizing lesions to the intra- or extradural and intra- or extramedullary spaces and to its spinal level, identifying herniated or bulging disks, and demonstrating the spinal cord in its entirety.

T1 weighting can be achieved on spin echo pulse sequences with a repetition time (TR) of ≤600 ms and an echo time (TE) of ≤20 ms respectively. Decreasing the TR below 600 ms will further improve the T1 contrast, but the trade-off is in loss of signal-to-noise ratio.[1] In addition, it is advantageous in axial imaging of the spine to image as much of the spine as possible. This requires a longer TR to obtain more slices, and the trade-off (if the number of data acquisitions is kept constant) is increased acquisition time and more susceptibility to motion artifacts.

On the other hand, TR can be reduced for sagittal images, since a fewer number of slices will cover the spine from one side to the other. Shortening the TR reduces the available number of slices. Decreasing the TE improves T1 contrast as well as the signal-to-noise ratio. However, below 10 to 15 ms the signal-to-noise ratio may be compromised because of bandwidth restrictions.[1]

On the sagittal view, the vertebral bodies have a slightly higher-signal intensity (and appear white) than the intervertebral disks (which appear gray) on T1-

(Text continues on page 72)

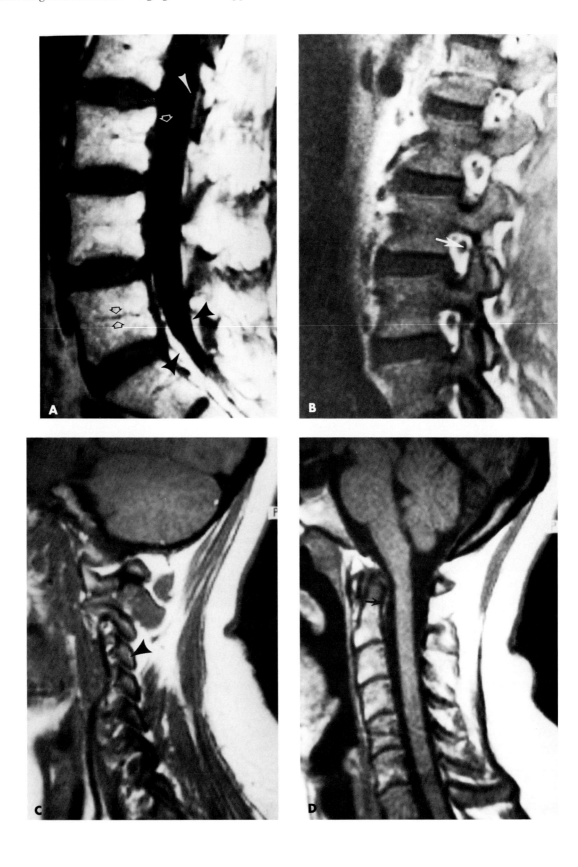

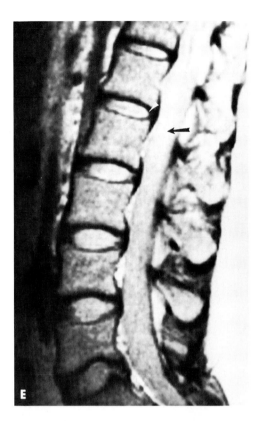

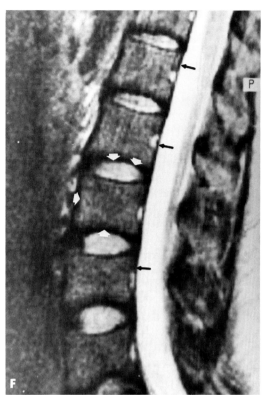

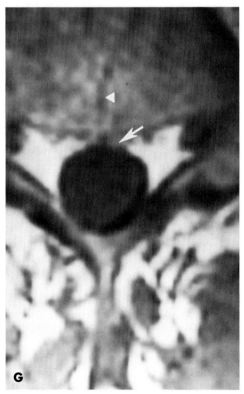

FIGURE 3–1. Normal anatomy of the spine (without contrast enhancement). **(A)** sagittal T1-weighted image of the lumbar spine with highest signal (white) from epidural fat (*black arrowheads*), then vertebral body (white), then disk and filum terminale (gray) (*white arrowhead*), and lowest signal from CSF (black) (*open white arrowhead*). The horizontal line of decreased signal in the center of the body is the bony canal of the basivertebral venous plexus (BVVP) (*open black arrowheads*). **(B)** Parasagittal T1-weighted image of the lumbar spine with epidural fat (white) highlighting keyhole configuration of the neuroforamen. The nerve root (*white arrow*) is seen as an ovoid structure within the epidural fat. **(C)** Parasagittal T1-weighted image of the cervical spine showing the facets (*black arrowhead*). **(D)** Sagittal T1-weighted image of the cervical spine showing the posterior longitudinal ligament to be isointense in signal with the spinal cord, blending with the tectorial membrane at the tip of the dens (*black arrow*). **(E)** Sagittal T2-weighted (balanced) image of the lumbar spine showing the annulus fibrosis of the disk as decreased signal (*white arrowhead*). The CSF (*black arrow*) appears isointense relative to the disk. **(F)** Sagittal heavily T2-weighted image of the lumbar spine shows the cortical bone as a black rim (*white arrowheads*) surrounding the vertebral body, and the posterior longitudinal ligament as a linear black structure (*black arrows*) along the posterior margins of the bodies. **(G)** Axial T1-weighted image of the cervical spine showing epidural fat as white and dural sac as dark gray. The site of the BVVP is seen as a defect within the center of the vertebral body (*white arrowhead*). The epidural venous plexus (*white arrow*) is isointense relative to the body (gray) and is located between the body and the dural sac.

weighted images (see Fig. 3–1). The signal intensity from the vertebral bodies should be relatively uniform. With age, the vertebral bodies may develop focal areas of increased signal intensity on T1-weighted images, representing fatty infiltrate, with characteristic decrease in intensity on the T2-weighted images, and endplate herniation of disk material representing Schmorl's nodes may occur. Bony islands also alter the normal homogeneous appearance of the vertebral bodies, appearing as areas of decreased signal intensity on T1-weighted images. Because of their sharp margins and lack of increased signal intensity on the T2-weighted images, bone islands can be differentiated from metastatic lesions. If there is a diffuse, infiltrative process in the marrow, a reversal in signal intensity may occur, with the intervertebral disks appearing brighter than the vertebral body on T1-weighted images.[2]

The epidural fat surrounds the dural sac in the lumbar region, appearing white on T1-weighted images, and is visualized both anteriorly and posteriorly on sagittal views. Laterally, the epidural fat within the neuroforamen has a teardrop configuration, with the exiting nerve root sleeve appearing as an ovoid structure of intermediate signal (see Fig. 3–1). There is less fat in the thoracic spine and even less in the cervical spine.

The facet joints are seen well in the lumbar and cervical region on more laterally located sagittal images (see Fig. 3–1). In the cervical region the posterior longitudinal ligament blends with the tectorial membrane and apical ligament, also being isointense relative to the spinal cord (see Fig. 3–1). The spinal cord is of intermediate-signal intensity and thus appears gray, contrasting sharply with black CSF.

On the axial view the intervertebral disk appears darker than the vertebral body and is separated from the dural sac by high-signal intensity epidural fat and by intervening Batson's vertebral venous plexus, which has an intermediate signal and thus appears gray. The posterior cortical defect where the basivertebral venous plexus enters the vertebral body may be seen in this view (see Fig. 3–1). The epidural fat extends into the neuroforamen allowing the latter structure to be well visualized.

T1-Weighted Contrast-Enhanced Imaging of the Normal Spine

Another important use of T1-weighted pulse sequences is for contrast-enhanced imaging with current contrast agents, which exhibit strong T1 relaxation properties (and weaker T2 relaxation enhancement). Although contrast is not used routinely for normal spinal imaging, the conspicuity of the cervical neuroforamen and the disk–dural sac interface are better defined,[3] particularly in the patient with very little epidural fat, and the disk–dural sac interface is enhanced in the lumbar spine by venous plexus enhancement.

On the sagittal views, the penetrating basivertebral venous plexus appears as a linear enhancing structure that pierces the vertebral body at its posterior cortex, midway between the endplates. The enhancing venous plexus is seen more consistently in the cervical and lumbar region anterior to the dural sac (Fig. 3–2). In the cervical region, the plexus is larger laterally, compared with the midline (see Fig. 3–2). The tectorial membrane (anteriorly and posteriorly) and the apical ligament may enhance in the cervical region (see Fig. 3–2). Enhancement of the venous plexus in the cervical region may improve visualization of the nerve roots within the foramen. The spinal cord does not enhance, nor do the intervertebral disks, unless reparative granulation tissue is present within the disk. In the latter situation, disk enhancement is delayed and may not be seen on immediate postcontrast MR studies.[4]

On the axial view in the cervical region, the exiting nerve root may become more conspicuous as the surrounding venous plexus in the foramen enhances (Fig. 3–3). The enhancement of the basivertebral vein within the vertebral body may occasionally be seen (see Fig. 3–3), as well as its site of penetration (Fig. 3–4). Enhancement of the nerve root ganglion may also be apparent in both the cervical and lumbar regions (Fig. 3–5).

T2-Weighted Spin Echo Imaging

T2-weighted pulse sequences are optimal for detection of intramedullary lesions, which will appear as areas of abnormal high-signal intensity, and for increasing the contrast between CSF–spinal cord and CSF–vertebral body interfaces. Because of its long T2 relaxation time, CSF appears white or bright and affords a myelographic-like picture on heavily T2-weighted images (see Fig. 3–1). Sagittal views are important for the same reasons discussed earlier for T1-weighted sagittal images. However, the conspicuity of the disk edge is better seen on the T2-weighted images, owing to the sharp contrast interface between the annulus fibrosis (which is hypointense or black on T2-weighted images, and demarcates the posterior margin of the disk) and CSF (see Fig. 3–1). Because of the long TR and TE required for T2-weighted spin echo images, which both make this type of scan more prone to motion artifacts, gradient echo images are often substituted.

T2-weighting can be achieved on spin echo pulse sequences with a long TR of 2 to 3 seconds, and most institutions utilize a double-echo technique. A short first echo (TEs of 25 to 45 ms) provides a proton density or mildly T2-weighted image with a high signal-to-noise ratio. On this scan, CSF has intermediate-

(Text continues on page 76)

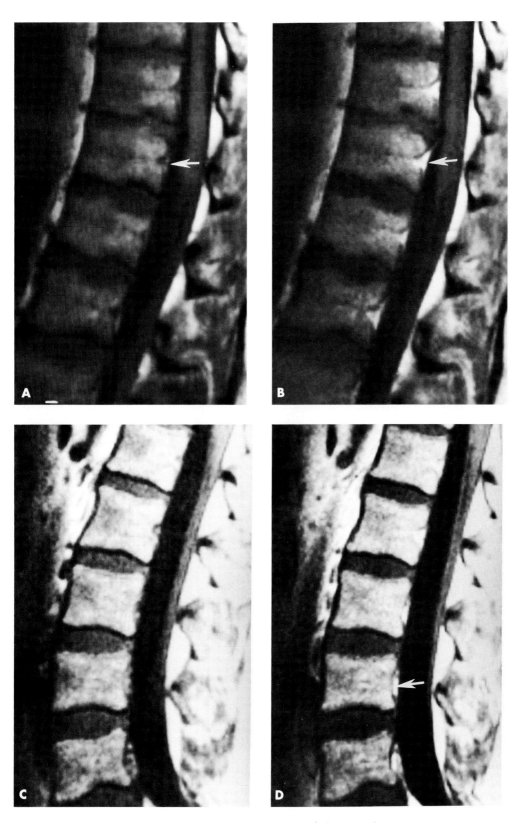

FIGURE 3–2. Pre- and postcontrast-enhanced MR images of the normal spine. **(B, D)** Post-gadopentetate dimeglumine; **(F, G)** post-gadoteridol. **(A)** Sagittal T1-weighted precontrast image of the thoracic spine. The site of penetration by the BVVP (*white arrow*) appears as a defect in the posterior cortical margin. **(B)** Postcontrast image corresponding to **A** showing enhancement of the BVVP (*white arrow*), within the thoracic vertebral body. **(C)** Sagittal T1-weighted precontrast image of the lumbar spine. **(D)** Postcontrast image corresponding to **C**, showing enhancement of the epidural venous plexus (*arrow*) behind the vertebral body. *(continued)*

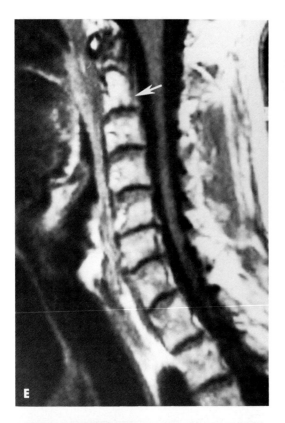

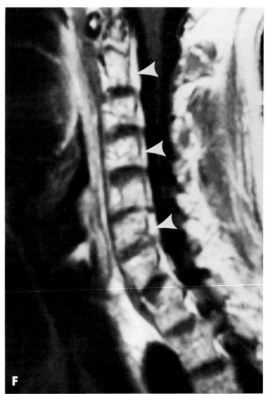

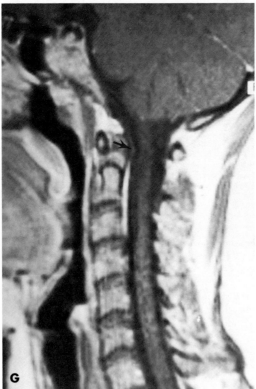

FIGURE 3–2 (cont.). (E) Parasagittal T1-weighted precontrast image of the cervical spine. The epidural venous plexus (*white arrow*) is gray or isointense relative to the cord. **(F)** Postcontrast image, corresponding to **E**, showing enhancing epidural venous plexus (*white arrowheads*), which is larger off the midline. **(G)** Postcontrast cervical spine image showing the enhancing tectorial membrane and apical ligament (*black arrow*) extending from the dens tip superiorly.

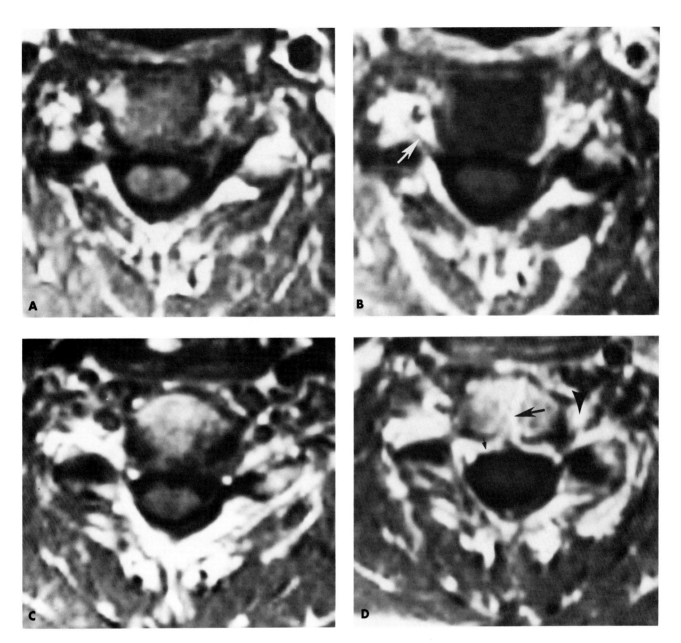

FIGURE 3-3. Pre- and postcontrast (gadopentetate dimeglumine) MR images of the normal cervical spine in the axial plane. **(A)** T1-weighted precontrast image of the cervical spine at the disk space level. **(B)** Postcontrast image, corresponding to **A**, which demonstrates the exiting nerve roots (*white arrow*) by enhancing the epidural plexus in the neuroforamen. **(C)** T1-weighted precontrast image of the cervical spine at the midvertebral body level. **(D)** Postcontrast image, corresponding to **C**, showing enhancement of both the epidural venous plexus (*small black arrow*), which now separates the dural sac from the body (compared with **C**); the basivertebral venous plexus (BVVP) (*large black arrow*), which penetrates the body in the center posteriorly and extends almost to the anterior cortex; and the vertebral arteries in the transverse foramina (*large black arrowhead*).

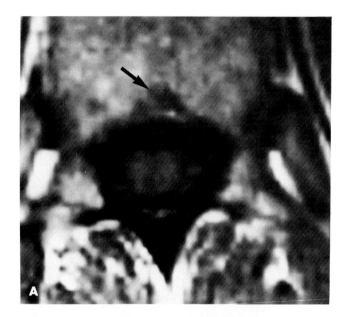

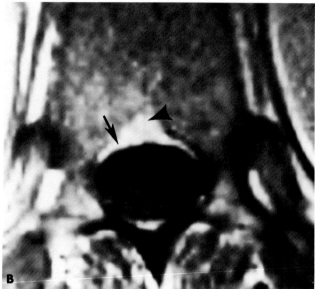

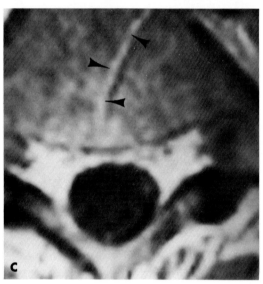

FIGURE 3–4. Pre- and postcontrast (gadopentetate dimeglumine) MR images of the normal thoracic spine in the axial plane. **(A)** Axial T1-weighted precontrast image of the thoracic spine. The penetrating BVVP is of intermediate-signal intensity (*black arrow*). **(B)** Postcontrast image of **A**, showing enhancement of epidural venous plexus (*black arrow*) and site of BVVP penetration (*black arrowhead*). **(C)** Postcontrast (gadoteridol) image in thoracic spine, at a different anatomic level (same patient as Figure 3–1), showing enhancement of BVVP within the body (*black arrowheads*).

signal intensity, allowing intramedullary lesions to be seen without being hidden by bright CSF signal intensity. A TE of 70 to 100 ms is typically employed for the second echo, providing a heavily T2-weighted image. Because of the intrinsically low signal-to-noise ratio on T2-weighted images, a reduced matrix (192 × 256) is often employed. There will be slight degradation in resolution along one axis. However, an additional benefit is the decrease in scan time compared with a square (256 × 256) matrix.

On the sagittal view, the vertebral bodies appear gray or hypointense relative to CSF (which appears white). The change in signal intensity of the vertebral bodies from white or hyperintensity on T1-weighted images to gray or hypointensity on T2-weighted images is characteristic of fatty tissue. The nucleus pulposus is hyperintense, compared with the vertebral body, be-

cause of its water content. The annulus fibrosus is hypointense relative to the nucleus pulposus and appears black (see Fig. 3–1). Cortical bone appears as a thin black rim surrounding the vertebra, and the posterior longitudinal ligament also appears black (see Fig. 3–1). The spinal cord appears gray and is highlighted by the surrounding CSF, which appears white.

Gradient Echo Imaging

Patients with spinal lesions generally have pain and are often unable to tolerate the relatively longer scan times of spin echo sequences (10 minutes). Motion occurs because of discomfort, degrading the quality of the MR images. Motion compensation techniques utilizing cardiac gating do not solve this problem because they add to the scan time. Gradient echo imaging helps consid-

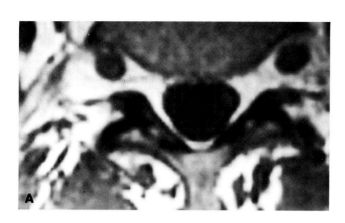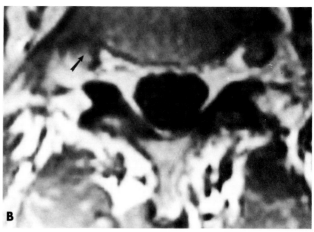

FIGURE 3–5. Contrast enhancement (gadoteridol) of the normal lumbar nerve root ganglion. **(A)** Axial T1-weighted precontrast image of the lumbar spine showing the nerve root ganglion lateral to the neuroforamina. **(B)** Postcontrast image of A, showing enhancement of the nerve root ganglion (*black arrow*) owing to fenestrated endothelium of the venous plexus in the neuroforamen.

erably because it attacks the problem of motion by faster data acquisition and, thereby, actually reduces scan times.

With gradient echo scans, the short TR considerably reduces data acquisition time, with T2 contrast maintained by employing a reduced flip angle. By definition, in gradient echo technique the 180° radiofrequency (rf) pulse is eliminated and signal echoes are generated by gradient reversals. With further modifications, it is even possible to obtain subsecond single-slice images.[5] However, in subsecond scanning the trade-off is either in resolution or in the signal-to-noise ratio.

Use of three-dimensional (3-D) acquisition in the cervical region may improve anatomic detail, particularly of the neuroforamen, since thinner slices (with reduction in partial volume effects) and contiguous slices (without the need for an interslice gap) can be obtained.[6] However, 3-D techniques can be more sensitive to patient motion, and "wraparound" (aliasing) artifacts occur.[7]

The most commonly employed gradient echo sequences are the FLASH (fast-low-angle-shot) short TR techniques known as FISP, FFE, FAST, CE-FAST, and GRASS. These techniques may be helpful if the patient is unable to tolerate long scan times. In many instances T2-weighted gradient echo techniques may be substituted in lieu of spin echo techniques. However, gradient echo techniques are very sensitive to magnetic susceptibility changes and may produce significant image artifacts, which are discussed later. Furthermore, the signal is not a true T2 signal, but rather a T2*, and may not be as useful in evaluating intramedullary lesions.[4]

Gradient echo techniques have been more sensitive than conventional spin echo imaging in evaluation of

extradural disease, especially for detecting prolapsed disks, but not for extruded disks.[8] Short TE (6 to 13 ms), short TR (200 to 300 ms), and small flip angles (10 to 20°) appear to be optimal for extradural disease, producing a myelogram-like picture and having the additional benefit of a short examination time. However, gradient echo techniques appear to be less sensitive for intradural disease, when compared with conventional T1-weighted spin echo images.[9] Others feel that a properly optimized gradient echo pulse sequence may replace spin echo imaging, particularly in the axial plane.[10]

Suggested imaging protocols for the cervical, thoracic, and lumbar spine are listed in the Appendix. A combination of T1- and T2-weighted spin echo and gradient echo sequences are employed. Electrocardiographic (ECG) gating is employed on T2-weighted spin echo sequences in the cervical and thoracic regions to minimize pulsation artifacts from CSF. The TR is typically set to be a multiple of the R-R interval on the ECG. To minimize artifacts from moving objects, such as the heart, aorta, lung, and abdominal viscera, rf pulses are applied to a "slab" of tissue in the coronal plane anterior to the spine. By saturating the protons in this tissue slab, motion artifacts originating from tissue within this coronal section will be minimized in the region of interest: the spine and its contents.

MECHANISM OF CONTRAST ENHANCEMENT

The current primary clinical MR contrast agents are extracellular gadolinium chelates, with the U.S. Food and Drug Administration (FDA) approval of gadopentetate dimeglumine (Gd-DTPA) in 1988. Two other contrast agents modeled after gadopentetate dimeglumine and nearing (or in) clinical use are gadoterate meglumine (Gd-DOTA; gadolinium tetraazacyclododecane tetraacetic acid) and gadoteridol [Gd-HP-D03A; gadolinium 1,4,7-tris (carboxymethyl)-10-(2'-hydroxypropyl)-1,4,7,10-tetraazacyclododecane]. The former has undergone extensive clinical trials in Europe, and the latter in the United States. Both of these newer contrast agents have a lower osmolality than gadopentetate dimeglumine. Furthermore, both have been utilized at higher clinical doses (up to 0.3 mmol/kg with gadoteridol).

Gadopentetate dimeglumine is composed of the gadolinium ion, a metal of the lanthanide series, the paramagnetic properties of which are due to its seven unpaired electrons, and a linear chelating agent (diethylenetriamine pentaacetic acid), the purpose of which is not only to reduce the toxicity of the metal but also to function as a carrier ligand. When bound by the chelate, gadolinium has one open coordination site (the other eight are bound) that permits fast exchange with bulk water molecules. The gadolinium ion is particularly effective in enhancing relaxation of hydrogen protons in water and, therefore, is important in proton MR imaging. Although gadopentetate dimeglumine affects both T1 and T2 relaxation rates, it is its effect upon T1 that is dominant at routine clinical doses and forms the basis for current T1-weighted contrast-enhanced MR studies.[11]

Enhancement of normal anatomic structures in the spine depends on the normal vasculature and whether or not the capillary endothelium is nonfenestrated (Batson's venous plexus) (see Figs. 3–2 to 3–4) or fenestrated (dorsal root ganglion, muscle, and marrow) (Fig. 3–5).[12] Nonfenestrated endothelium, such as occurs in the cerebral vasculature, confines the contrast agent to the intravascular space. Therefore, contrast enhancement reflects the interaction between the contrast agent and water molecules within the blood vessels. Fenestrated endothelium allows the contrast agent to pass through the capillary walls into the interstitial space where it influences the relaxation properties of water molecules within the tissue. The net result is T1 shortening, and enhancing structures appear white or have increased signal intensity on T1-weighted pulse sequences. The normal spinal cord itself has not been reported to show enhancement.[12]

Enhancement of pathologic processes in the spine depends on whether there is breakdown of the normally intact blood–tissue barrier (intramedullary lesions), with the resulting T1 relaxation enhancement occurring within the interstices of the spinal cord lesion, or alteration of vascularity (extramedullary lesions) with T1 relaxation occurring within abnormal blood vessels or tissue.[13] Preliminary experiences suggest that the patterns of contrast enhancement encountered may aid in differential diagnosis, although definitive tissue typing cannot be made. Since spinal pathology traditionally has been classified as intradural (intramedullary and extramedullary) and extradural, it is useful to divide the discussion of the patterns of abnormal contrast enhancement similarly.

PATTERNS OF ABNORMAL CONTRAST ENHANCEMENT

In intradural–intramedullary lesions, for example, neoplastic disease, the location and homogeneity (or lack of) of the enhancement aids in differential diagnosis similar to contrast-enhanced CT scans. Contrast-enhanced MR studies are better able to define the margins of the tumor, separate tumor from edema or syrinx, and highlight areas of cystic changes or necrosis. It is important for surgical purposes to pinpoint tumor and differentiate it from accompanying edema, which may also enlarge the cord.

An intense, homogeneous pattern of enhancement, with sharp margins in an intramedullary lesion, tends to favor an ependymoma. In addition, this tumor may be multinodular and tends to occupy the entire spinal cord. Whereas enhancement in a more irregular fashion, with less well-defined margins, favors astrocytoma, which tends to grow in an infiltrative manner. All astrocytoma types appear to enhance with paramagnetic contrast, even low-grade tumors. However, overlap in the pattern of enhancement occurs so that a definitive diagnosis cannot be made.[13]

A strongly enhancing, solid tumor nidus within a large area of syrinx should suggest a hemangioblastoma. These tumors, like astrocytomas, tend to infiltrate the cord and produce an irregular pattern of contrast enhancement, with poorly differentiated margins. However, a tumor nidus within an area of edema may also be seen with metastasis to the spinal cord.[13]

Other lesions, such as multiple sclerosis plaques, have been reported to enhance with contrast, but the experience is too limited to characterize the pattern of enhancement. Contrast enhancement has not been reported with cavernous hemangiomas in the cord. Subacute (which can mask enhancement) and chronic hemorrhage, with crescentic areas of high-signal intensity mixed with low-signal intensity are seen in association with cavernous hemangiomas.[13] Just as with intracranial plaques, a lesion that enhances within the spinal cord indicates an active multiple sclerosis (MS) plaque. Delayed enhancement of the spinal cord because of ischemia and infarction has been reported in cases with arteriovenous fistulas.[14]

In intradural–extramedullary lesions, contrast enhancement likewise better defines the abnormality and allows differentiation from the spinal cord. Because of the extramedullary location, tumors have an obtuse angle relative to the cord, compared with an acute angle seen with an intramedullary lesion. The myelographic principles of intramedullary versus extramedullary lesion differentiation can also be applied to MR imaging of the spine. The abnormal enhancement seen with these lesions is due to abnormal vascularity.

Intense, homogeneous, sharply marginated enhancement favors either a meningioma or a nerve sheath tumor. Both tend to be isointense compared to the spinal cord on precontrast T1-weighted images. Nerve sheath tumors tend to be high intensity on T2-weighted images, and meningiomas have only a slightly higher intensity.[13] Neurofibromas, in particular (which can be both intradural and extradural), have a somewhat characteristic appearance, with strong signal intensity on T2-weighted images. Unlike astrocytomas, meningiomas and nerve sheath tumors are clearly outside the spinal cord. However, these tumors may appear to project within the spinal cord on just one view. Therefore, as with myelography, it is important that two, preferably orthogonal, views (axial and sagittal, but coronals may be obtained in addition) are obtained.

So-called drop metastases are well visualized with contrast-enhanced MRI. Multiple, nodular and sheetlike lesions are characteristic. Multiple, tortuous, dilated enhancing vascular structures are typical for an arteriovenous malformation (AVM). However, a similar appearance can be noted on the unenhanced T2-weighted MR images because of flow voids. Contrast enhanced MR imaging may not add further to the evaluation of an AVM unless spinal cord infarction or ischemia is present.

In extradural lesions, contrast-enhanced MR imaging plays little role, with the exception of degenerative disk disease and in the differentiation of postoperative fibrosis from recurrent herniated disk. The majority of lesions in this category tend to be bony, either secondary (metastatic involvement) or primary, with encroachment on the spinal canal. Contrast may even mask the presence of metastasis by enhancing the lesion to the same intensity as that of fatty marrow. Contrast-enhanced MR imaging may play a role in the evaluation of soft-tissue extensions of primary bone tumors by better defining their margins. It has been reported to have little role in the evaluation of arachnoiditis.[15] However, in infections of the spine, contrast-enhanced MR imaging may be important not only in the detection but also in evaluating the extent of the infection.

Enhancement is seen immediately postcontrast in most of the clinically described lesions. Intradural–extramedullary lesions have been reported to have the most prominent early enhancement. Extradural lesions also show immediate enhancement. In intramedullary,

extramedullary, and extradural lesions, delayed imaging showed a slight increase in the degree of enhancement. Necrotic tumors may be better imaged with delayed postcontrast studies.[16] Rapid gradient echo imaging has been performed in meningiomas, showing a striking and immediate uniform uptake of contrast.[13]

Quantification of the degree of enhancement does not aid in differentiation of tumor from normal tissue or distinguishing the various types of tumor. Tumors were reported to show increases of 70% to 350%, and epidural scar, normal venous plexus, and dorsal root ganglion had 200% enhancement. Schwannomas tended to enhance more than astrocytomas or ependymomas, but not consistently.[16]

An imaging strategy for contrast agent use in the evaluation of a suspected spinal abnormality is outlined in Table 3–1, with the applications listed in decreasing order of importance. However, this scheme may change as other contrast agents are approved for routine clinical use at higher doses.

Pitfalls and Artifacts

A common pitfall in conventional spin echo MR spine imaging is caused by truncation artifacts that alter the size of the spinal cord and canal as well as produce a syrinxlike artifact projecting within the spinal cord. These artifacts are produced as the result of Fourier transforms used to reconstruct MR images, and occur in the direction of the phase-encoding gradient.[17] Because of frequency encoding of each row of data within the imaging matrix, the data are represented as waves. In regions of abrupt signal change that produces a sharp step in the intensity, such as occurs at the bone–CSF and CSF–spinal cord interface, the oscillatory nature of these waves produces an overshoot and undershoot of signal intensity. Each peak represents high-signal intensity or a bright band, and each valley

Table 3–1 Indications for Contrast-Enhanced MR Imaging of the Spine

Major Indications

Intramedullary spinal tumors
Extramedullary spinal tumors
Metastasis (osseous and soft-tissue component)
Drop metastasis
Postoperative fibrosis versus recurrent herniated nucleus pulposus
Inflammatory (diskitis and abscess)
Vascular lesions (AV malformations)
Multiple sclerosis

Minor Indications

Degenerative disk disorder
Trauma
Congenital lesions other than tumor or vascular malformations
Improving visualization of the interface between the dural sac and disk

represents decreased signal intensity or a dark band. The maximum overshoot occurs at 0.5 pixel from the interface, and maximum undershoot occurs at 1 pixel.

The Gibb phenomenon states that the overshoot will always persist no matter if even an infinite Fourier series is used with an amplitude of 9% over or under the ideal intensity value. In the strictest sense, this phenomenon refers only to the first peak or fluctuation. The oscillatory effect, which is called the Gibb phenomenon, is also known as the edge-ringing or ring artifact. Since Fourier transforms cannot be infinite, the data are truncated, giving rise to the term truncation artifact.

The pseudosyrinx effect is well recognized on sagittal images of the cervical spine, occurring in the direction of the phase encoding. On T1-weighted images, since CSF is black, a dark truncation band is seen exactly 4 pixels behind the CSF–spinal cord interface. This produces a dark band centrally within the spinal cord on sagittal images, which may be mistaken for a syrinx. Likewise, on the T2-weighted images a bright truncation band is seen that may also resemble a syrinx. Since the cervical spinal canal size is normally 7 to 16 pixels and the spinal cord size even smaller, and the artifact occurs 4 pixels behind the CSF–spinal cord interface, the truncation band is most noticeable within the cord. In the thoracic region because the canal and cord are larger, this effect is not as noticeable.[17]

On routine spin echo axial imaging, this artifact is not as apparent. Therefore to verify the presence of a syrinx, the suspect abnormality should be seen on axial images. However, if gradient echo techniques are employed in the axial plane, with a 256×128 matrix and phase encoding in the anteroposterior direction, an artifactual central spinal cord syrinxlike picture can be produced.

Truncation artifacts also produce edge enhancement at high-contrast interfaces. This will cause edges, such as cortical bone, to appear thicker, raising the question of spinal stenosis. Edge enhancement does not improve anatomic definition and may actually cause blurring. This may result in pseudoatrophy of the spinal cord. Pseudoatrophy may further be enhanced by manipulation of the photographic window width and level.[18]

The most commonly recommended method for reducing truncation artifact is to use a smaller pixel, either by using a larger matrix (256×256) or decreasing the field of view (surface coil). This does not eliminate the artifact, but rather, increases the number of band artifacts over a given area. However, the intensity and width of the bands decrease and, accordingly, are not as evident on the final images. The Gibb phenomenon cannot be eliminated, even if one could perform an infinite Fourier series.[17]

Changing the phase-encoding direction (for sagittal imaging) to the longitudinal direction (cephalocaudad) will eliminate the ring artifact across the spinal cord. However, the artifact is now projected onto the bodies and disks as horizontal bands. The trade-off is that CSF is not as dark, the CSF–cord margins are blurred, and wraparound artifacts may occur.

An increase in the number of phase-encoded steps can minimize the effects of truncation artifacts, but the trade-off here would be increasing the data acquisition time, thereby making the images more prone to detail loss from motion.

Postprocessing filtering of the raw data has also been applied. These are mathematical filters, the purpose of which is to remove high-frequency data. Filters known as the "Hamming" window or "triangular" window do not eliminate the primary overshoot and undershoot, but rather, the secondary waves. Unfortunately, since the data are smoothed and the slopes of the waves are flattened, there can be image blurring and loss of spatial resolution.[17]

Chemical-shift artifacts occur at fat–water interfaces, producing an apparent edge enhancement, with an alternating band of dark and bright signal. This may be mistaken as an area of abnormal contrast enhancement on axial images, particularly when a clinical history suggestive of drop metastasis or arachnoiditis is provided.[19]

Another recently reported spin echo artifact occurs with residual oily based intrathecal contrast medium (Pantopaque), employed for previous myelography, which on T1-weighted imaging may mimic a spinal lipoma. Chemical shift occurs at the oil–CSF interface, which may mimic the dura, falsely localizing the oily contrast to the epidural compartment.[20]

A significant pitfall occurs with gradient echo-imaging techniques, which are commonly utilized in lieu of T2-weighted imaging of the spine because of the decreased scan time. Artifacts are caused by the magnetic susceptibility differences occurring at bone–soft tissue interfaces in the spine. This results in distortion and, actually, enlarges bone margins, especially if long TEs are used. In cervical spondylosis, this can produce the artifactual appearance of spinal canal stenosis, as well as that of neuroforaminal stenosis.

Tsuruda studied the effects of magnetic susceptibility and motion on cervical spine phantoms utilizing a 3-D gradient echo technique.[21] With longer TE, the gradient echo images overestimated the degree of neuroforaminal stenosis when compared with CT. In addition, motion mimicked osseous hypertrophy, which further contributed to overestimation of the degree of foraminal stenosis. He recommended using the shortest possible TE.

Magnetic susceptibility effects are also pronounced at air–tissue interfaces, especially at the sphenoid sinus where the effect can be readily recognized as an area of signal dropout. The susceptibility effect is less pronounced at bone–tissue interfaces and appears as exaggeration or elongation of bony spurs leading to incorrect assessment of canal size.[22]

Even if short echo times are used with gradient echo imaging to reduce the magnetic susceptibility artifact in spinal imaging, the canal size is more accurately assessed on CT scans. If surgical decompression or foraminotomy is being considered, it may be prudent to obtain a CT scan as well.

DEGENERATIVE DISK DISEASE

Degenerative disease of the spine is the sequelae of aging and is manifested by degeneration of the intervertebral disk, with loss in height, disk bulging or herniation, osteophytic bony formation narrowing either the spinal canal or neural foramen, hypertrophic facet changes, and subluxation or displacement of the vertebral bodies. Depending on the area and degree of involvement, degenerative disease is manifested clinically as pain or neurologic changes, either neurosensory or motor weakness.

Traumatic injury to the spine, neoplasia, neurodegenerative disorders, metabolic diseases, hematologic disorders, postradiation changes, and certain congenital disorders may accelerate the degenerative changes. It is not in the scope of this chapter to discuss the pathophysiology of degenerative disease of the spine or the full scope of its manifestations, but rather to emphasize changes that are best evaluated by contrast-enhanced MR imaging, those related to disk degeneration.

The intervertebral disk consists of a central nucleus pulposus and surrounding annulus fibrosus. The disk is of intermediate-signal intensity and appears gray on T1-weighted images (see Fig. 3–1). Because of the high water content of the nucleus pulposus and the inner annulus, these structures have high-signal intensity on T2-weighted images, and the outer annulus fibrosus appears as a concentric ring of low-signal intensity (see Fig. 3–1).[23]

With aging, the disk desiccates and loses its water content. The hydrostatic pressure decreases internally, resulting in collapse and thinning of the disk as well as loss of its high-intensity signal on T2-weighted images (Fig. 3–6). Type II collagen increases in the annulus, and both it and the nucleus pulposus lose as much as 70% of the water. The cartilaginous endplates become thinned, and fissuring of the annulus and nu-

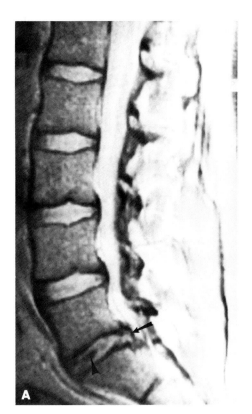
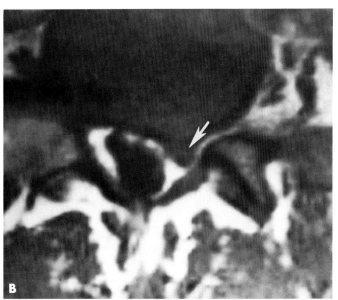

FIGURE 3–6. L5–S1 herniated disk. **(A)** Sagittal T2-weighted MR image of a herniated disk (*arrow*) at the L5–S1 level. There is decreased signal (*arrowhead*) from the disk caused by loss of water content from the nucleus pulposus. **(B)** Axial T1-weighted MR image of an L5–S1 herniated disk (*arrow*), which is of slightly higher-signal intensity than CSF within the dural sac.

cleus occurs, with attempts at regeneration producing granulation tissue. Tears of the annulus fibrosus can be detected with contrast T1-weighted MR images as linear areas of enhancement within the disk. Experimental data indicate that it is the granulation tissue within the fissures that is enhancing.[23]

Corresponding changes occur in the vertebral marrow adjacent to the disk space, giving rise to three patterns described by Modic.[23] Type I changes consist of decreased signal intensity in the marrow on T1-weighted sagittal images, and increased signal intensity on T2-weighted images. Type II changes consist of increased signal intensity on T1-weighted images, and isointense to slightly increased intensity on T2-weighted images. Type III changes consist of decreased signal intensity on both T1- and T2-weighted images. Neither of the first two types of changes correspond with endplate sclerosis on plain radiographs, whereas the third type does.[23]

With degeneration of the annulus fibrosus, either bulging or herniation of the nucleus pulposus can occur. Bulging disks have an intact annulus fibrosus that bulges outward along with the nucleus in a centrifugal fashion, generally symmetric, but occasionally unilateral. Herniated disk protrudes through a rent in the annulus fibrosus and exhibits a characteristic MR appearance of higher-signal intensity; the nucleus pulposus protrudes through the lower-signal intensity annulus with a dumbbell or narrow waist appearance (see Fig. 3–6). With an extruded disk, the nucleus has completely herniated through the annulus, but remains in contiguity with the central nucleus pulposus. In a sequestered disk, the nucleus pulposus fragment is not only completely herniated through the annulus rent, but is completely separated from the central nucleus and may migrate inferiorly or superiorly to the disk space or into the neuroforamen (Fig. 3–7). Herniated disk fragments have intermediate intensity on T1-weighted images and intermediate- to high-signal intensity on T2-weighted images. However, sequestered disk fragments may exhibit an intermediate- or low-signal intensity on T1-weighted images, with high-signal intensity characteristic on T2-weighted images (see Fig. 3–7). A thin black rim along the posterior edge of the herniated disk may be seen; this may represent either posterior longitudinal ligament, a portion of the annulus fibrosus, or calcification.[23]

In addition to the reparative changes that occur within the intervertebral disk, similar changes may occur along the posterior edge of the herniated disk material. Peridiskal scar tissue formation in the anterior epidural space can occur in the virgin spine (Fig. 3–8). Histologically, it has an appearance similar to postoperative scar tissue, consisting of vascularized tissue, with a large extracellular space and collagen fibers that may sequester paramagnetic contrast agent.[3] It is this scar tissue that allows contrast-enhanced MR imaging to play a role in the evaluation of disk herniation. Peridiskal scar enhancement is intense and improves conspicuity of a herniated disk (see Fig. 3–7).

Disk herniation is less common in the cervical region, partly because it is not subject to the weight bearing that occurs in the lumbar region, and because the uncinate processes provide additional buttressing for the nucleus pulposus along the posterolateral margins. Degenerative spurs are more common in the cervical region with aging, as are uncinate spurs that produce foraminal narrowing and, thereby, nerve root compression.

Before the advent of MRI, thoracic disk herniations were considered to be rare. They tend to be asymptomatic, but the incidence has recently been reported to be as high as 15%.[24] A thoracic disk herniation appears to have the same signal characteristics as the native thoracic intervertebral disk, although its periphery tends to have a low-signal intensity and may be difficult to distinguish from CSF on T1-weighted scans. This may be related to the presence of calcification or spurs, which are occasionally seen on CT.[25]

Lumbar disk herniations tend to be eccentric because the posterior longitudinal ligament is centrally located and absent laterally (see Fig. 3–6). A disk herniation may also be entirely within the neuroforamen, the so-called lateral herniated disk, which may not be detected by myelography.

In the cervical and thoracic regions where epidural fat is less, or in the patient with very little epidural fat in the lumbar region, it is often difficult to distinguish an intervertebral disk from the dural sac, especially when there is diffuse disk bulging. This problem is even more pronounced in the cervical region where not only is the canal smaller, but also truncation artifacts and magnetic susceptibility effects are more noticeable, degrading spatial resolution and blurring the bone–CSF interface. Contrast-enhanced MR imaging may play a minor role in this situation.

Contrast enhancement of Batson's vertebral venous plexus and the cervical venous plexus increases the contrast difference between the disk and the dural sac or nerve roots by enhancing the interposed venous plexus (which is low-signal intensity on nonenhanced T1-weighted MR imaging) (see Figs. 3–2 and 3–3). This improves the assessment of canal and foraminal stenosis and separates the diffusely bulging disk from the dural sac. In addition, with disk herniation and compression of the venous plexus, there is dilatation of the veins both above and below the level of herniation. Contrast enhancement of the venous plexus increases the conspicuity of the herniated disk, especially in the

(Text continues on page 85)

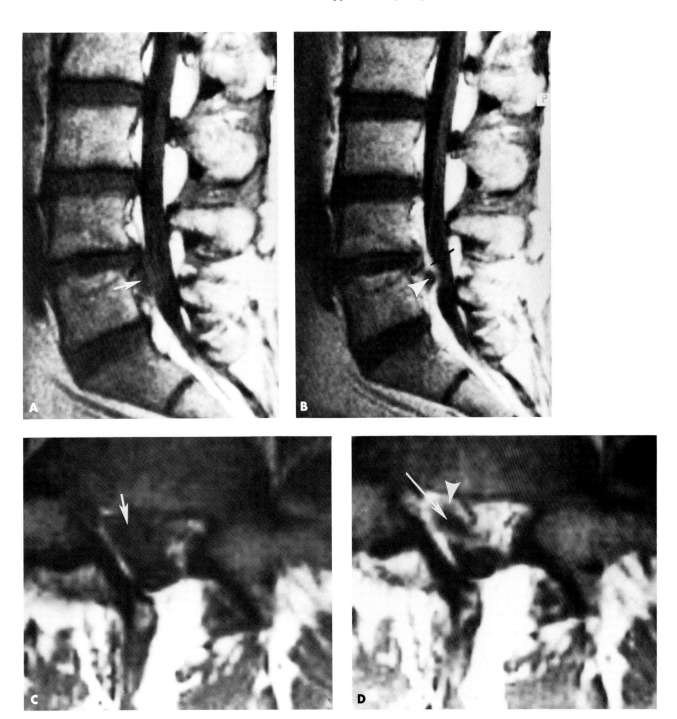

FIGURE 3–7. Postoperative scar versus recurrent disk. **(A)** Precontrast sagittal T1-weighted MR image of a postoperative L4–5 herniated disk with recurrence and a free fragment (*arrow*) located inferior to the disk space level. **(B)** Postcontrast (gadopentetate dimeglumine) sagittal T1-weighted MR image of **A**, showing peridiskal scar enhancement (*arrow*) as well as the sequestered or free fragment recurrent disk (*arrowhead*). The conspicuity of the disk has been increased following contrast injection. **(C)** Precontrast axial T1-weighted MR image of **A**, showing soft-tissue intensity (*arrow*) in the canal on the right side at the L4–5 level, as well as the left laminectomy defect. **(D)** Postcontrast (gadopentetate dimeglumine) axial T1-weighted MR image of **C**, showing peridiskal scar enhancement (*arrowhead*) and the sequestered disk fragment (*long arrow*) as decreased signal intensity that does not enhance. Contrast enhancement of the scar increased the conspicuity of the free disk fragment.

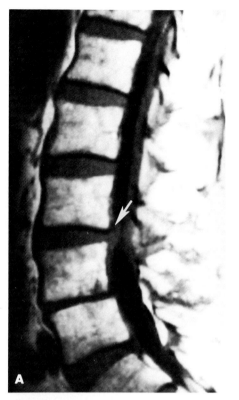
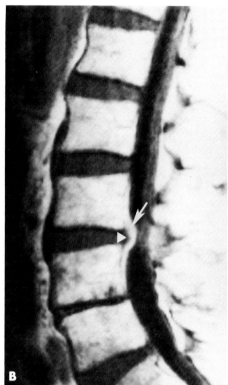
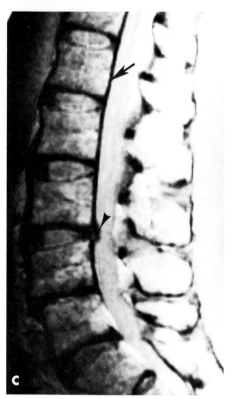

FIGURE 3–8. Peridiskal scar enhancement. **(A)** Precontrast T1-weighted MR image of a postoperative L4–5 disk with no surgery at the L3–4 level. Probable herniated nucleus pulposus (HNP) seen at the L3–4 level as an isointense mass (*white arrow*). **(B)** Postcontrast (gadopentetate dimeglumine) T1-weighted MR image of **A**, showing a definite L3–4 HNP (*arrowhead*) plus intense peridiskal scar enhancement (*arrow*). No scar or recurrent HNP is present at the L4–5 level. **(C)** Sagittal T2-weighted MR image of **A**, showing intact posterior longitudinal ligament as a black line (*black arrow*) and the peridiskal scar at L3–4 as irregular low-signal intensity along the posterior edge of the disk (*black arrowhead*).

cervical region. Contrast-enhanced MR imaging probably has a more important diagnostic role when degenerative changes, with hypertrophic bone formation, are present and, consequently, is more important in the elderly patient.

We have recently instituted the use of contrast enhancement in the routine evaluation of the lumbar and cervical spine at our institution. In a review of 100 lumbar MR examinations, the use of contrast enhancement had a significant positive impact on the economic cost of workup for herniated disk.[26] The addition of an MRI contrast agent eliminated the need for further myelography and CT, resulting in a lower overall cost to the patient. Contrast was most helpful when motion was present and when diffusely bulging disks and paucity of epidural fat made the distinction between disk and sac difficult. In a few cases, the noncontrast MR examination had ruled out a herniated disk, which was subsequently found on the contrast-enhanced study. The herniated disk was mistaken for a bulging disk on the noncontrast study. The disk and sac conspicuity is significantly improved in the cervical region because of the more prominent epidural veins. In addition, the cervical nerve roots are consistently well seen owing to enhancement of the foraminal venous plexus. Contrast-enhanced T1-weighted MR imaging may become the method of choice for foraminal stenosis evaluation, since it is not plagued with the problems of gradient echo imaging.

Postoperative Lumbar Spine

A commonly encountered clinical problem is continued or recurrence of back pain after surgery, the so-called failed back surgery syndrome.[27] Of the multiple causes for this syndrome, including recurrent herniated disk, epidural fibrosis, arachnoiditis, lateral recess and spinal canal stenosis, mechanical instability (facet subluxation), and iatrogenic (surgical nerve root injury, incorrect operative level), contrast-enhanced MR imaging plays a major role in the evaluation of the first two. It is very important to make the distinction between postoperative fibrosis and recurrent disk herniation because, in the former, repeat surgery will not alleviate the symptoms and may worsen them by creating more scar tissue. Myelography, postmyelographic CT scanning, and intravenous contrast-enhanced CT scanning have had limited success in differentiating scar from recurrent disk.

The appearance of the spine on unenhanced MR imaging after surgery has been well documented and, at times, differentiation between postsurgical fibrosis and recurrent herniated disk can be made. The level

of the surgery can be easily identified if a laminectomy has been performed, with absence of bone on T1-weighted images (see Fig. 3–7), and soft-tissue edema manifested on both T1-weighted (heterogeneous intermediate-signal intensity) and T2-weighted (high-signal intensity) images in the immediate postoperative period. There is disruption and asymmetry in the muscle–fat planes posteriorly. The dural sac may also bulge posteriorly, if the laminectomy defect is large enough. However, if a laminotomy with microsurgery techniques has been performed, the tissue disruption may be minimal, with absence of the ligamentum flavum being the only recognizable finding.[28]

In the immediate postoperative period, the rent or disruption of the annulus through which the herniation of the nucleus pulposus occurred can be seen best on T2-weighted images. Edema in the immediate postoperative period obliterates the normal high-signal intensity from the epidural fat on T1-weighted images. This renders the fat–dural sac interface indistinct. In the immediate postoperative period, edema has intermediate-signal intensity on T1-weighted and increased signal intensity on T2-weighted images at the site of the original disk herniation, so that it appears that the original herniation is still present, with mass effect on the dural sac on both sagittal and axial views. Unlike the preoperative MR images, the high-signal intensity on T2-weighted sagittal and axial images from the nucleus pulposus blends with the CSF following surgery. The loss of the CSF–disk interface is due to surgical disruption of the annulus fibrosus, which has a low-signal intensity on T2-weighted images.[28]

Postoperative hemorrhage can also occur, exhibiting the characteristic T1 and T2 changes of hemoglobin. In the subacute period, the high-signal intensity changes of blood degradation products may actually improve contrast differentiation between the dural sac and adjacent edema.

After 2 to 6 months, healing occurs and the MRI appearance changes. The tear in the annulus becomes less apparent or disappears. On T1-weighted sagittal images, the bulging or protrusion of the nucleus becomes less but occasionally may appear unchanged compared with the preoperative study. However, on the T2-weighted sagittal images, the horizontally oriented high-signal intensity, representing herniated nucleus, is replaced with a vertically oriented high-signal intensity along the posterior rim of the disk representing anterior epidural fibrosis. This anterior scar is similar in appearance to the anterior epidural scar on spines with herniated disks that have not been surgically treated. The relative lack of change makes unenhanced MRI of the postoperative spine unreliable in the 2-month period after surgery.[28]

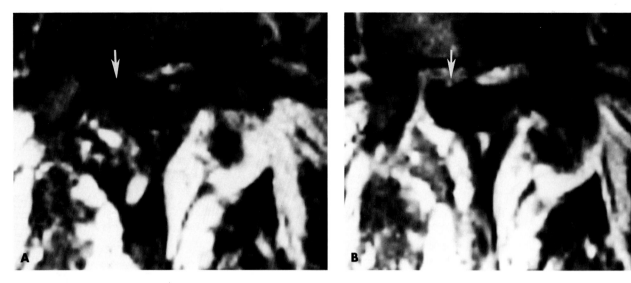

FIGURE 3–9. Postoperative fibrosis. **(A)** Precontrast axial T1-weighted MR image at L4–5 performed to rule out a herniated disk in a patient with previous surgery at this level. Scar tissue appears black (*arrow*) on the right side and is indistinguishable from the dural sac. **(B)** Postcontrast (gadopentetate dimeglumine) T1-weighted MR image of **A**, showing that the previously black-appearing scar has now enhanced (*arrow*). There is no mass effect on the dural sac.

After 2 years or more, scar tissue tends to have intermediate- to low-signal intensity, whereas immature scar may have a higher-signal intensity, probably related to the presence of granulation tissue and increased vascularity on T2-weighted images (Fig. 3–9). The low-signal intensity in old scar is similar to the MRI characteristics of collagenous or compact fibrous tissue.[29]

Morphologic changes and, to a lesser degree, signal intensity changes allow differentiation of scar from recurrent disk on nonenhanced MRI, with a degree of accuracy similar to IV contrast-enhanced CT scanning. Recurrent herniated disk exhibits mass effect as well as contiguity with the central nucleus, unless there is a free fragment, and is smoothly marginated (Fig. 3–10), whereas scar tissue does not exhibit mass effect (unless very large), usually conforms to the epidural space without compressing the dural sac, may even cause retraction of the sac toward the scar, and has irregular and poorly defined margins (see Fig. 3–9).[28] Recurrent herniated disk is of isointense to slightly increased intensity on T1-weighted images and does not exhibit as high a signal intensity as scar tissue on T2-weighted images (see Fig. 3–9). Scar tissue, on the other hand, has hypo- to isointensity and intermediate- to high-signal intensity on T1- and T2-weighted images, respectively. Free fragments have very high signal intensity on T2-weighted images.

Unfortunately, discrimination between scar and recurrent disk without the use of a contrast agent is based mainly on interpretation of T2-weighted images, which have poorer signal-to-noise ratios than T1-weighted images. Furthermore, because of the longer acquisition times for T2-weighted images, the studies are often prone to poor resolution because of motion, since it is recurrent pain that brings the patient back for more studies.

Since scar tissue enhances consistently and contrast-enhanced MR studies have been shown to be 96% accurate, contrast media clearly have a major role in the differentiation of scar from recurrent herniated disk.[30] In addition, since T1-weighted techniques are used, the signal-to-noise ratio is greater, and the images are less prone to motion artifacts. Contrast-enhanced MRI has been shown to be superior to contrast-enhanced CT scans in the differential diagnosis of recurrent herniated disk versus scar formation.[31]

It is the formation of scar tissue and the diagnosis of its presence that is the key element in contrast-enhanced MR imaging (see Figs. 3–8 and 3–9). Normally, disk material does not demonstrate contrast enhancement, whereas scar tissue consistently enhances heterogeneously on immediate postinjection scans, and more homogeneously on delayed scans. However, in delayed (30 to 45 minutes) imaging, disk material can also be seen to enhance. Therefore, it is important in the differentiation of scar from recurrent herniated disk that imaging be performed immediately after contrast injection.[11,28]

The mechanism of scar enhancement is related to the presence of vascularized tissue within the scar. Numerous capillaries within a stroma of collagen are present within scar tissue. It is presumed that the con-

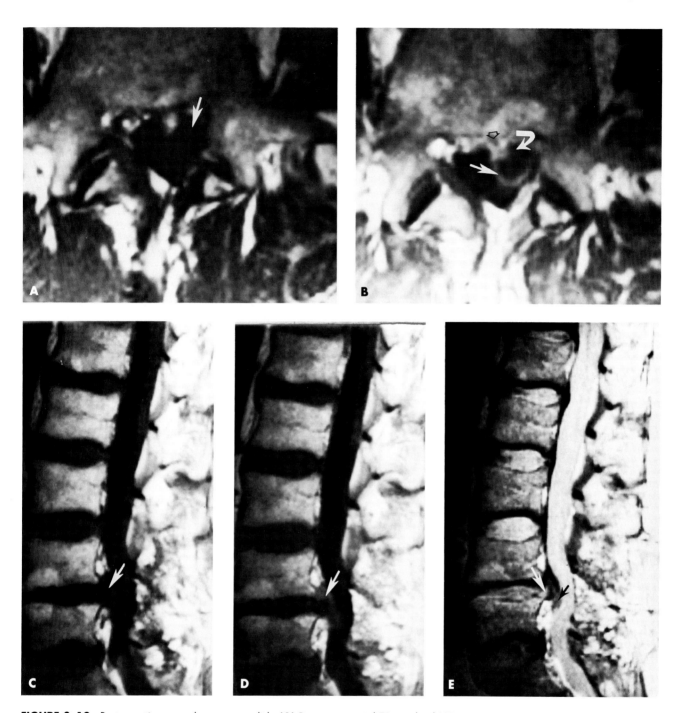

FIGURE 3–10. Postoperative scar plus recurrent disk. **(A)** Precontrast axial T1-weighted MR image of a postoperative patient at the L4–5 level, showing a soft-tissue mass (*arrow*) on the left side virtually indistinguishable from CSF within the dural sac. **(B)** Postcontrast (gadopentetate dimeglumine) T1-weighted MR image of **A**, showing recurrent HNP with mass effect (*curved arrow*) on the dural sac and peridiskal scar enhancement of the disk edge (*straight arrow*) increasing its conspicuity. There is also abnormal enhancement anterior to the recurrent disk, representing the site of annular rent (*open arrowhead*). **(C)** Precontrast T1-weighted sagittal MR image of **A**, with recurrent disk and scar tissue indistinguishable (*arrow*). **(D)** Postcontrast (gadopentetate dimeglumine) T1-weighted MR image of **C**, showing slight enhancement of scar (*arrow*) posterior to the recurrent disk, which shows no enhancement (compare with **B**, which is the same patient, but in the axial projection). **(E)** Sagittal T2-weighted MR image of the same patient showing scar as having a *lower* signal (*black arrow*) than the recurrent HNP (*white arrow*). Note that on the T2-weighted image the recurrent disk can be differentiated from the more irregular-margined scar tissue posteriorly.

trast material leaks out through the capillary walls, where it is sequestered within the collagenous extracellular space. On the other hand, disk material is less vascular.[4,32]

Peridiskal enhancement, which probably represents peridiskal scar formation, may be seen (see Fig. 3–10).[11,32] Alternatively, this could represent epidural venous plexus enhancement. The delayed contrast enhancement of the disk itself may be of some aid in differentiating disk fragments from nerve roots, since the latter do not enhance on delayed imaging.[30] The enhancement within the disk may be due to either scar formation or ingrowth of vascularity into the disk space.[33]

Scar tissue can be classified by location as anterior, lateral, or posterior. Anterior epidural scar in the virgin and operated-on back is similar histologically and in the pattern of contrast enhancement. Anterior scar always enhances, however long after surgery.[32] Lateral scar exhibits characteristics similar to anterior epidural scar, but not as consistently. Experimentally, posterior epidural scar (both in terms of imaging characteristics and histologically) is different from anterior scar.[34,35] In the postoperative period, the degree of contrast enhancement decreases after a 4-month period, rather than persisting as with anterior scar.

There may also be enhancement at the site of annular rent (see Fig. 3–10). At surgery in these cases, the thecal sac was reported to be tacked down to the rent. The authors felt that scar formation, with its associated vascularity, may be responsible for the enhancement at the rent.[28]

Bundschuh and associates obtained scar tissue from ten patients with failed back surgery syndrome and examined the tissue by light and electron microscopy.[36] They correlated the degree of contrast enhancement from CT and MR scans with the location of scar, its age, and its tissue characteristics.

Anterior epidural scar, which was felt to be younger, showed the most intense enhancement, followed closely by lateral epidural scar. The looser the gap junction in the capillary endothelium, and the larger the extracellular space, the more intense the enhancement.[36] Young scar had more loose junctional gaps, permitting contrast to leak out. The larger extracellular space with young, anterior epidural scar had more bulk water with which the contrast can interact, producing a stronger signal enhancement than would occur with smaller extracellular spaces.

Young scar or granulation tissue had very few micropinocytotic vesicles, a higher rate of luminal occlusion of vessels, and a lower blood perfusion rate, which would tend to decrease the degree of scar enhancement. In fact the vascularity in older, more mature scar would tend to favor more delivery of contrast and,

accordingly, more scar enhancement should be observed. However, this was not the case, leading Bundschuh and co-workers to conclude that vascular density is not a determining factor in terms of the degree of scar enhancement.

They concluded that intensity values alone did not help differentiate scar from recurrent herniated disk. Since herniated disk can also have granulation tissue, disk may enhance as well. Because of this overlap, they felt that both contrast-enhanced CT and MRI have an accuracy of only 80% in differentiating recurrent disk from scar.[36]

The typical changes of diskitis on MRI morphologically resemble those encountered on plain radiographs and CT scans. There is loss in height of the intervertebral disk, with irregular margins of the vertebral endplates. Loss in height may be difficult to assess, since there normally is some loss following surgical removal of a disk. Progressive loss in the height of the disk with an abnormal soft tissue mass is indicative of an active inflammatory process. Decreased intensity on T1-weighted images, and increased signal intensity on T2-weighted images of the endplates are seen with diskitis. However, the latter finding is to be distinguished from a normal finding of increased signal in the disk without loss in height, with a central horizontal line of decreased signal intensity on T2-weighted sagittal images. The central line represents an intranuclear cleft, with the decreased signal intensity caused by fibrous tissue (which develops within fissures). The presence of an intranuclear cleft allows the changes of normal aging to be differentiated from the inflammatory changes of diskitis.[37]

Postcontrast MR studies may demonstrate enhancement of the inflammatory mass (Fig. 3–11). However, it may be difficult to differentiate this enhancement from postoperative fibrosis and postsurgical changes. Contrast administration may also aid in the identification of an associated abscess, which should enhance (see Fig. 3–11).

Postoperative Cervical Spine

Because of differences in surgical technique for cervical compared with lumber diskectomy, the MR appearance is distinctly different. Diskectomy in the cervical region involves an anterior approach, drilling through the disk space. Bone graft is then placed into the disk space to provide stabilization. This graft has a variable appearance on T1-weighted images, depending on the marrow fat content. With solid bony fusion, the disk space disappears and the marrow appears contiguous between the two adjacent vertebrae.

Because of the drilling techniques employed, either microscopic bony or metallic fragments can produce

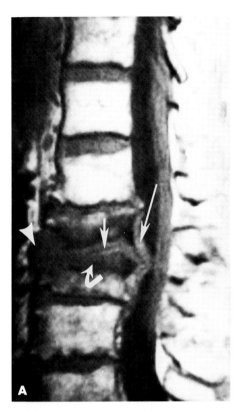
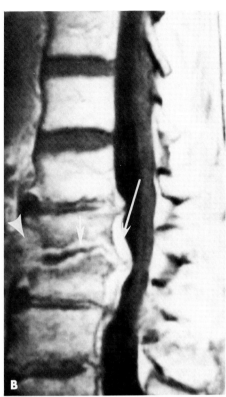
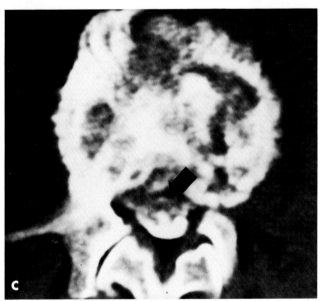

FIGURE 3-11. Postoperative (4 months after surgery) diskitis and abscess formation, with *Staphylococcus aureus* cultured from the disk space. A 54-year-old patient who presented with back pain and low-grade fever 1 month after diskectomy. An MRI was performed 3 months later because of persistent pain, despite antibiotic therapy. **(A)** Precontrast sagittal T1-weighted MR image of the lumbar spine showing at the L2–3 level marked loss in disk height and irregularity of the endplate (*white arrow*), as well as decreased signal intensity from the adjacent vertebral bodies (*curved arrow*). There is a soft-tissue mass anteriorly (*arrowhead*). There is also a markedly thickened posterior longitudinal ligament or possible anterior epidural scar (*long white arrow*). Patient with proved diskitis and osteomyelitis who developed an anterior abscess. **(B)** Postcontrast (gadopentetate dimeglumine) T1-weighted MR image of **A**, showing striking enhancement (*long white arrow*) of anterior epidural scar (or less likely thickened longitudinal ligament), and lesser enhancement of the endplates (*white arrow*) and anterior abscess (*arrowhead*). **(C)** Postmyelogram CT of the same patient demonstrating extensive bony endplate changes. The thickened posterior longitudinal ligament or anterior epidural scar (*black arrow*) is seen in front of the dural sac.

magnetic susceptibility artifacts with signal intensity dropout. These artifacts are much more evident on gradient echo imaging. If small enough, the artifact may be mistaken for an epidural defect, such as a bony spur.[28]

TRAUMATIC INJURY

Conventional T1- and T2-weighted sequences have been used, predominantly without contrast administration, in the evaluation of acute and chronic injuries to the spinal cord.[38,39] Contrast-enhanced MR imaging may have little role in the assessment of traumatic spinal cord imaging. However, spinal cord ischemia and infarction due to arteriovenous fistulas have been reported to enhance with contrast.[14]

Schouman-Claeys and colleagues produced a spinal cord injury model in dogs, but did not find any enhancement of the cord after injection of gadoterate meglumine (Gd-DOTA).[40] However, Casselman and coworkers demonstrated abnormal enhancement of the anterior portion of the spinal cord in a patient with anterior spinal artery occlusion resulting from a hyperflexion traumatic injury of the cervical spine.[41]

NEOPLASIA

Intramedullary

Cell types of tumors involving the spinal cord are similar to intracranial tumors. Intramedullary tumors are less common than extradural or intradural–extramedullary tumors. In general, larger proportions of intramedullary tumors are identified in children than in adults, compared with the other spinal locations.[42] Spinal cord tumors are from 3 to 12 times less common than primary cerebral tumors.[43] The symptoms from intramedullary tumors result from direct interference with the intrinsic structures of the spinal cord.

The role of contrast material is diverse for intramedullary neoplastic disease. Its application in neoplastic disease is primarily for localization of breakdown in the blood–brain barrier. This area of enhancement may be used to direct surgical biopsy and may also improve lesion detection. Magnetic resonance imaging is clearly more accurate in delineation of intramedullary lesions than any antecedent imaging modality. When combined with contrast material, evaluation of cystic change, mass effect, and inflammatory disease of the spinal cord has been dramatically changed by MRI. Additionally, the pattern of enhancement may also be used to follow the progress of therapy (Fig. 3–12).[44] Reliable identification of necrotic areas in tumors is possible following intravenous contrast administration.

In the setting of a complex syrinx, the neoplastic site may frequently be identified by the enhancement. The entirety of the syrinx should be scanned in both sagittal and axial planes for identification of the underlying neoplastic site.[45]

The differential diagnosis for intramedullary lesions primarily includes astrocytomas and ependymomas with additional considerations including hemangioblastomas and metastatic disease. Astrocytomas and ependymomas account for slightly over 90% of intramedullary tumors, with considerable overlap in appearance, making differentiation, at times, impossible. The general incidences of intramedullary tumors have been reported as 61% for ependymomas and 33% for either lower- or higher-grade astrocytomas.[46]

Ependymomas are most common in the lower thoracic cord and cauda equina, and the age, at presentation, is slightly older than cord astrocytomas. However there is a wide variation in the ages at presentation of both astrocytomas and ependymomas. They are also commonly found in the cervical region (Fig. 3–13). Myxopapillary cell types are a more benign variety and compose 27% to 30% of conus and filum ependymomas (Fig. 3–14),[47,48] and have been described to present with subarachnoid hemorrhage. Spinal ependymomas rarely calcify, in contrast with intracranial ependymomas. They tend to occupy the entire width of the cord, which is consistent with centrifugal expansion away from the ependymal cells of the central canal.[13] Eccentrically located lesions are less likely to be ependymomas. They usually intensely and uniformly enhance with contrast agents on T1-weighted sequences.[13]

Astrocytomas are most commonly found in the cervical canal and upper thoracic region. They tend to be more eccentric in location, relative to the central canal. Similar to most spinal cord tumors, they display decreased signal intensity on T1-weighted images and increased signal intensity on T2-weighted scans. When located in the spinal cord, they are usually lower-grade tumors. However, there is a greater propensity for enhancement of spinal cord gliomas, compared with intracranial gliomas of similar grades (Fig. 3–15).[13,49,50] Astrocytomas may enhance in a more patchy, irregular pattern than that observed with ependymomas,[13] with concomitant cord enlargement at the site of the tumor. The full extent of the tumor may not be delineated by contrast enhancement; hence, a T2-weighted examination should also be obtained to further delineate the neoplastic process.[50] Delayed enhancement may be seen with necrotic tumors. Neoplastic cysts usually have foci or regions of enhancement. Cysts that are cranially or caudally located to the tumor are usually

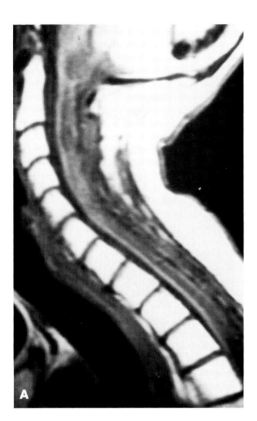

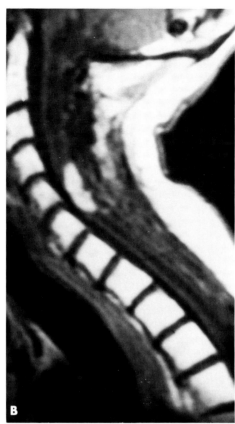

FIGURE 3-12. Recurrent ependymoma. **(A)** T1-weighted sequence displays high-signal intensity throughout the marrow, consistent with prior radiation therapy. Postsurgical changes are identified in the lower cervical spine. **(B)** Postcontrast (gadopentetate dimeglumine) scan reveals enhancement consistent with recurrent ependymoma.

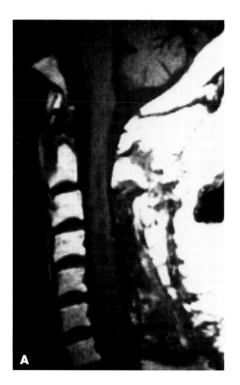

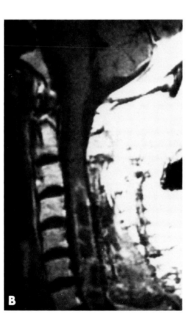

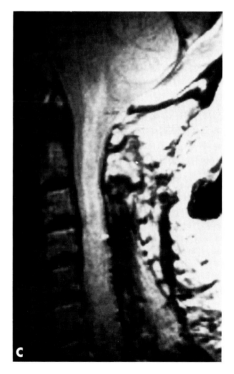

FIGURE 3-13. Ependymoma. **(A)** T1-weighted sagittal scan demonstrates expansion of the upper cervical cord with a central region of decreased signal intensity. **(B)** Postcontrast (gadoteridol) T1-weighted sagittal scan reveals peripheral enhancement, with central necrosis or cystic changes. **(C)** The T2-weighted examination less accurately identifies the epicenter and internal characteristics of the tumor. (Courtesy of Dieter Schellinger, MD and Mark J. Carvlin, PhD)

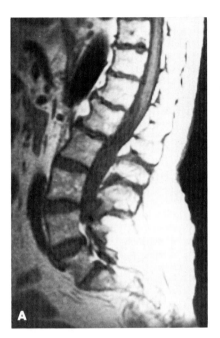
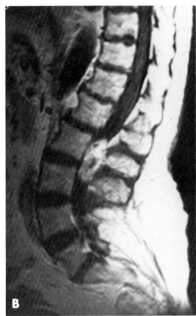
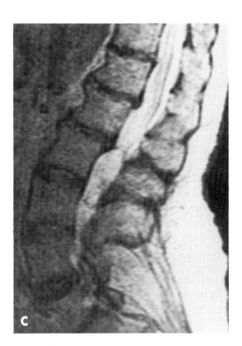

FIGURE 3–14. Myxopapillary ependymoma of the filum. **(A)** T1-weighted sagittal scan reveals a questionable abnormality at L-2 and L-3. **(B)** The postcontrast scan (gadoteridol) eloquently displays the tumor. **(C)** It is difficult to identify the mass on the T2-weighted sequence. (Courtesy of Adam E. Flanders, MD)

benign.[51] Higher-grade astrocytomas of the cord, similar to higher-grade intracranial astrocytomas, may display CSF seeding.

There is intense enhancement of hemangioblastomas following intravenous contrast administration. They constitute about 3% of cord tumors. There is an especially high prevalence of hemangioblastomas in patients with von Hippel–Lindau disease (Fig. 3–16). They may be multiple throughout the cord with this disease and have a high vascular flow rate, with enlarged vessels simulating an arteriovenous malformation (AVM).

Metastatic involvement of the cord may occur by drop metastases (Fig. 3–17) or direct vascular seeding. Contrast is particularly useful for evaluation of metastatic disease. Small drop metastases that involve only the pial surface can be reliably detected only by MRI following contrast enhancement with thin-section imaging. Preferably, both sagittal and axial planes should be obtained. Higher-grade gliomas and primitive neuroectodermal tumors (i.e., medulloblastomas, pineoblastomas) are the most common tumors that give rise to drop metastases. Lung, breast, and prostate carcinoma, as well as lymphoma and leukemia, have also been identified to involve the leptomeninges on contrast-enhanced MR scans.[52] Neoplastic seeding of the CSF pathways may cause diffuse leptomeningeal enhancement.

Intramedullary metastases are usually associated with significant vasogenic edema. Clinically, there is rapid progression of symptoms, as opposed to primary cord tumors that are more insidious. The edema, at times, may involve a large segment of the spinal cord.[51] The contrast-enhanced scan can more accurately identify the underlying lesion.[51] Lung and breast carcinoma and melanoma are the most common histologic types.

Intradural–Extramedullary

The most common types of neoplasia in this category are meningiomas, schwannomas, and neurofibromas; although, some drop metastases could be classified in this group. These tumors usually markedly enhance, a characteristic related to the absence of the blood–brain barrier. Contrast-enhanced MR scans appear to be equivalent to the myelogram–CT examination for detection of lesions in this category. Contrast-enhanced MR scans have been reported to detect intradural–extramedullary lesions routinely as small as 3 mm and, occasionally, as small as 2 mm (Fig. 3–18).[53] Leptomeningeal spread along nerve roots may occasionally be more accurately identified on contrast-enhanced MR scans than on myelogram–CT.[53] However, the CT–myelogram combination is probably more accurate for evaluating more focal disease. The use of CSF cytologic techniques exceeds both contrast-enhanced MRI and myelogram–CT studies in detecting the presence of lep-

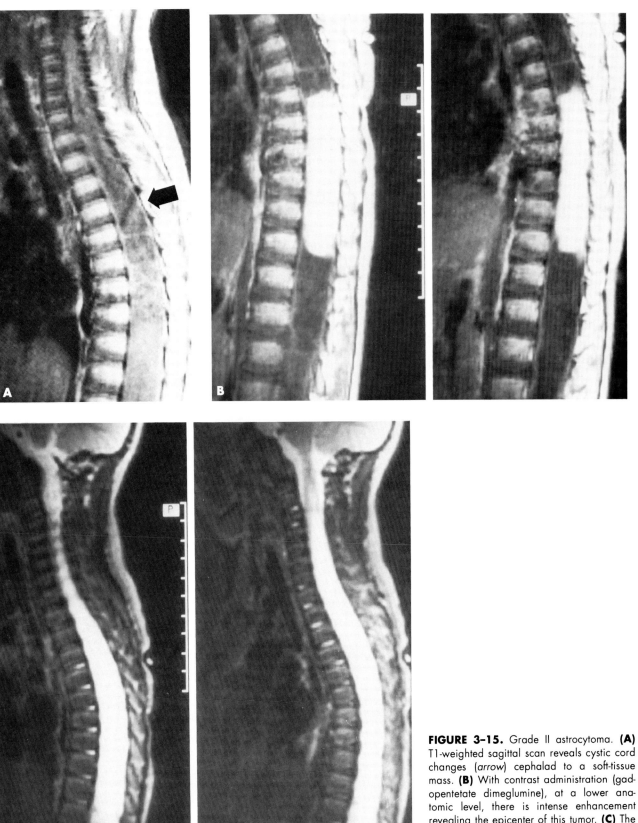

FIGURE 3-15. Grade II astrocytoma. **(A)** T1-weighted sagittal scan reveals cystic cord changes (*arrow*) cephalad to a soft-tissue mass. **(B)** With contrast administration (gadopentetate dimeglumine), at a lower anatomic level, there is intense enhancement revealing the epicenter of this tumor. **(C)** The T2-weighted scan provides little additional information.

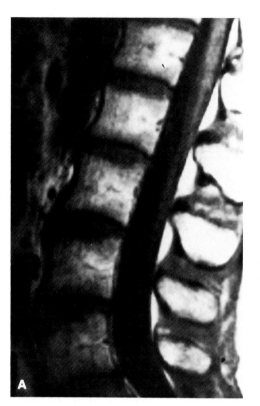
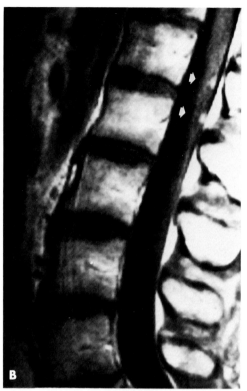

FIGURE 3–16. Multiple hemangioblastomas in a patient with von Hippel–Lindau disease. **(A)** T1-weighted sagittal examination displays a normal-appearing conus. **(B)** There are two small hemangioblastomas (*arrows*) identified on the postcontrast (gadopentetate dimeglumine) scan adjacent to the lower thoracic cord and conus.

tomeningeal seeding.[53] Contrast-enhanced MR scans are far superior in detection of small lesions, compared with routine T1 and T2 sequences, since the signal intensities of these lesions frequently approach that of CSF.

Meningiomas, typically, display homogeneous enhancement (Fig. 3–19). They are most commonly located in the thoracic spine and, occasionally, cervical spine (Fig. 3–20) and anterior foramen magnum. Involvement of the lumbar spine is rare. Meningiomas are usually located laterally or posterolaterally where the roots converge to exit the canal. They may also occur along the pial surface. They are more common in middle-aged women and are usually benign, slow-growing tumors.

Schwannomas intensely enhance and appear to enhance to a greater degree, on the average, than intramedullary gliomas,[54] but they frequently have a nonhomogeneous enhancement pattern. Small schwannomas or neurofibromas may be difficult to detect without contrast material, but can be very symptomatic. They tend to occur in a slightly younger population than meningiomas and are slow-growing lesions that expand the neuroforamen (Fig. 3–21). They are usually

solitary. Schwannomas have a tendency to involve the dorsal sensory nerve root, although some motor ones are reported. In contrast, neurofibromas encompass or incorporate the ganglion or nerve. Lumbar roots are most commonly involved, with frequent involvement as well of both cervical and thoracic roots. They, rarely, may be intramedullary when associated with neurofibromatosis. They are both intradural and extradural in 15% of cases, whereas the majority (58%) are intradural–extramedullary (Fig. 3–22). Extradural schwannomas are seen in 27% of cases.[55] Malignant forms of schwannomas may also be seen.

Leptomeningeal "seeding" from systemic tumors is similar to intracranial metastases in incidence, with lung and breast carcinoma having the highest prevalence. Of all intracranial tumors, medulloblastoma (PNET), glioblastoma multiforme, oligodendroglioma, and ependymoma have the highest incidence of drop metastases.

The lumbosacral region is the most common location for leptomeningeal seeding when the spinal canal is involved.[56] This may be related to gravity effects and CSF flow patterns.[56] There may be a multifaceted pattern of enhancement, with nodular masses most com-

(Text continues on page 97)

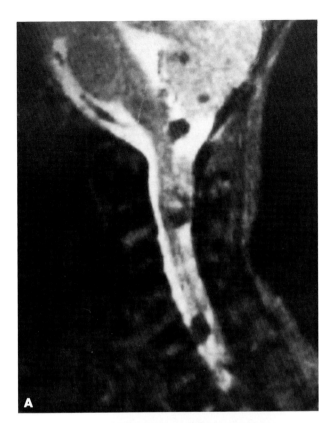

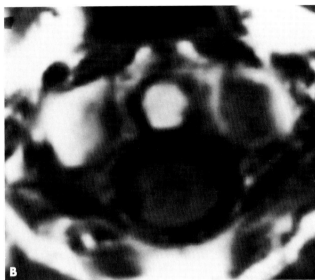

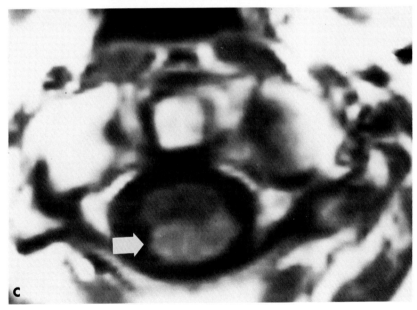

FIGURE 3-17. Drop metastases from a primitive neuroectodermal tumor. **(A)** The T2-weighted scan displays decreased signal intensity within multiple lesions caused by hemosiderin deposition. **(B)** Axial precontrast T1-weighted image reveals an enlarged cord. **(C)** The postcontrast (gadopentetate dimeglumine) scan separates the spinal cord at this level from a dorsal soft-tissue mass (*arrow*), which demonstrates slight enhancement.

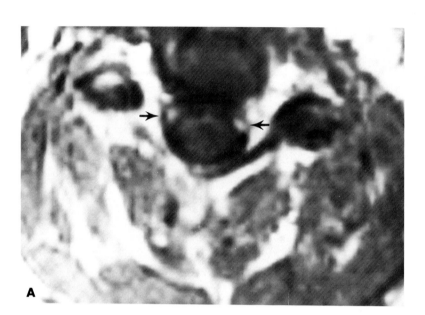

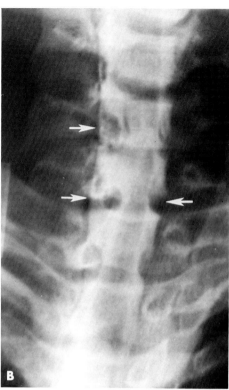

FIGURE 3–18. Leptomeningeal seeding from a myoblastoma originating at the conus. **(A)** Axial postcontrast (gadopentetate dimeglumine) T1-weighted sequence in the cervical spine reveals two small enhancing lesions associated with the exiting nerve roots (*arrows*). **(B)** Magnified and collimated images from a cervical myelogram display multiple small lesions adjacent to the cervical roots. A complete block was discovered at the level of the conus. The primary lesion was demonstrated by MRI (not shown) at the level of the conus.

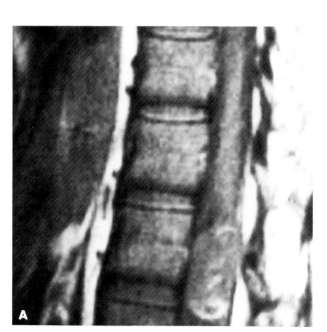

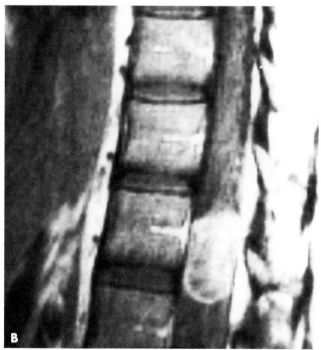

FIGURE 3–19. Meningioma at the level of the conus. **(A)** Sagittal precontrast T1-weighted examination reveals the lesion adjacent to the conus. **(B)** Following contrast administration (gadopentetate dimeglumine) there is moderate enhancement of the lesion.

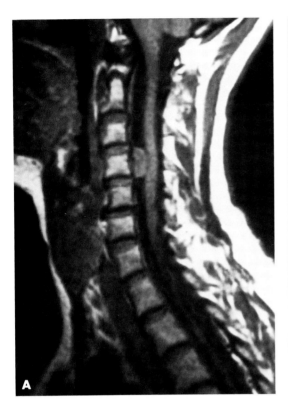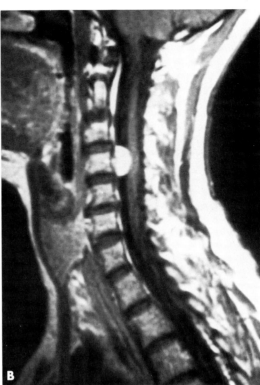

FIGURE 3-20. Meningioma. **(A)** Precontrast T1-weighted sequence displays the lesion anterior to the cord at C-4. **(B)** Following contrast administration (gadoteridol), there is intense and uniform enhancement. (Courtesy of Kenneth R. Maravilla, MD)

monly seen, but occasionally there may be uniform leptomeningeal spread (Fig. 3–23) or, rarely, complete filling of the subarachnoid space.

Extradural

Magnetic resonance imaging offers a less invasive method for evaluating the spine for cord impingement caused by extradural lesions. Contrast enhancement, although not routinely necessary, may more accurately delineate the extradural component of the process.

Metastatic disease is the most common tumor causing extradural cord impingement. Other than hemangiomas, all other primary bone tumors are less commonly seen and infrequently cause spinal impingement.

The primary role of contrast enhancement in the extradural compartment is for identification of the soft-tissue component of the tumor, particularly in the epidural space if there is a paucity of fat. Also, contrast material is helpful in differentiating disk herniation from epidural tumor. A biopsy of vertebral lesions that enhance may improve diagnostic yields.[57] Tumor enhance-

ment may yield information concerning response to therapy similar to nuclear medicine bone scans.[57]

Contrast enhancement is of less value in the evaluation of metastatic disease[12,58,59] limited to bone, owing to the normal high-signal intensity of marrow on T1-weighted sequences. Enhancement may actually make the metastatic lesion less conspicuous (Fig. 3–24). However, fat-suppressed scans may ameliorate this problem. There can be different degrees of enhancement of different lesions in the same patient. Enhancement of vertebral bony lesions is quite variable. In patients with normal marrow, T1-weighted images are highly accurate in identifying tumor involvement.[57,60] Contrast enhancement frequently decreases conspicuity of lesions within vertebral bodies; however, in the elderly population or for patients with heterogeneous marrow, contrast enhancement may improve the recognition of metastatic disease.

Metastatic disease may cause spinal impingement in 5% of patients with a disseminated neoplastic process. A report of frequencies of involvement is thoracic, 69%; lumbar, 16%; and cervical, 15%.[61]

(Text continues on page 101)

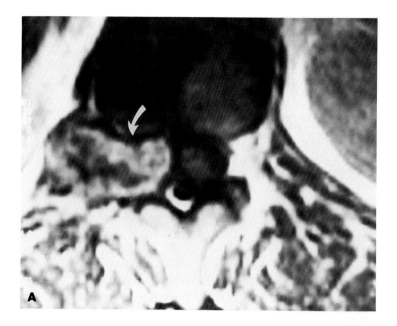

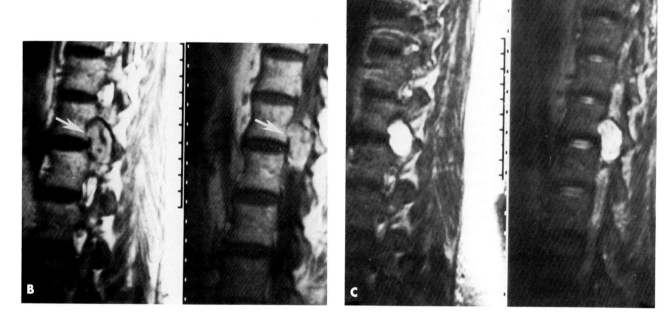

FIGURE 3–21. Schwannoma expanding the right T11–12 neuroforamen. **(A)** The T1-weighted axial examination following intravenous administration of contrast material (gadopentetate dimeglumine) demonstrates inhomogeneous enhancement of the lesion (*curved arrow*), which extends into the paraspinal soft tissues. **(B)** The postcontrast sagittal T1-weighted scan delineates the mass involving the neuroforamen (*arrows*). **(C)** T2-weighted images well depict this high-signal intensity lesion.

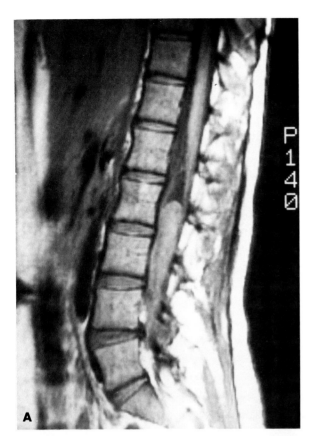

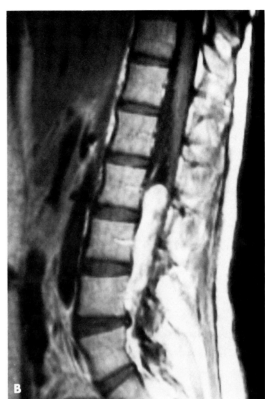

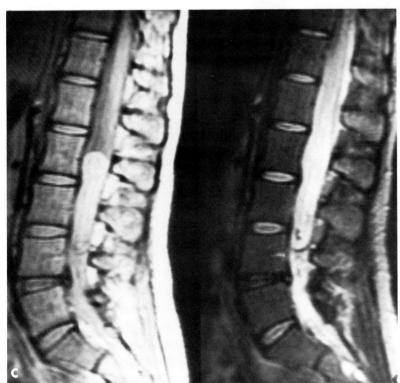

FIGURE 3–22. Intradural schwannoma. **(A)** There is a large mass involving the cauda equina in the lumbar spinal canal. **(B)** Following contrast administration (gadoteridol), there is intense enhancement. **(C)** The second echo of the T2-weighted series less readily delineates the mass. (Courtesy of Michael A. Mikhael, MD)

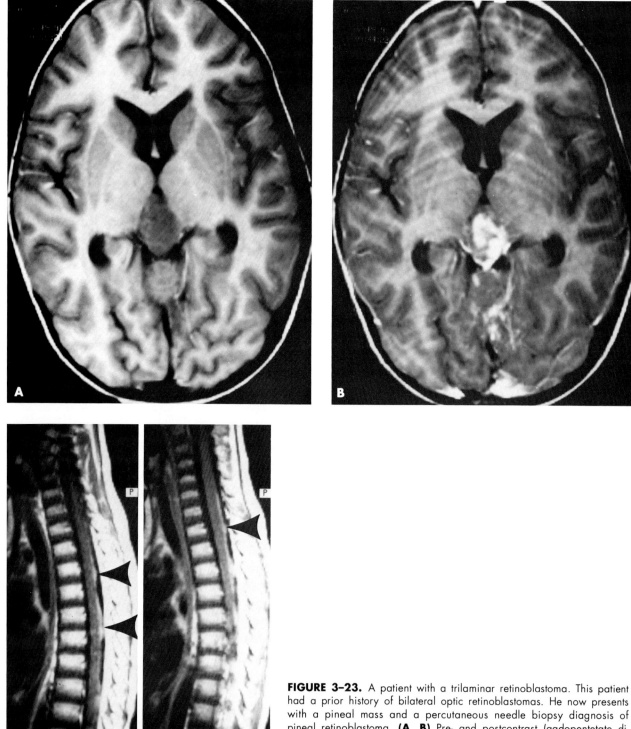

FIGURE 3-23. A patient with a trilaminar retinoblastoma. This patient had a prior history of bilateral optic retinoblastomas. He now presents with a pineal mass and a percutaneous needle biopsy diagnosis of pineal retinoblastoma. **(A, B)** Pre- and postcontrast (gadopentetate dimeglumine) T1-weighted scans identify the enhancing pineal mass. **(C)** Postcontrast T1-weighted scans display uniform coating of tumor over the leptomeninges of the lower cervical and thoracic cord surfaces. There is a propensity for greater involvement of the dorsal cord surface (*arrowheads*).

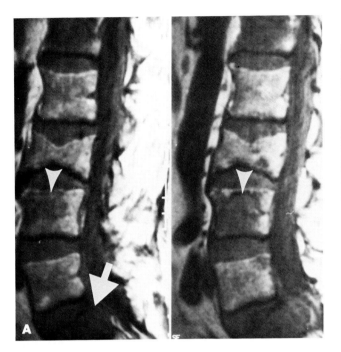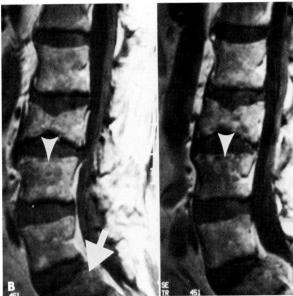

FIGURE 3–24. Metastatic disease involving the bony spinal canal. **(A)** The T1-weighted sagittal spin echo scan readily depicts the marrow replacement by the metastatic lesions (*arrows*). **(B)** The lesions are less conspicuous on the postcontrast (gadopentetate dimeglumine) scan (*arrows*). Note that the disk spaces are of similar signal intensities, reflecting similar "centering" and "windowing" of the scans.

The role of contrast material in primary tumors of bone is similar to that in metastatic disease.[62] Vertebral hemangiomas are seen in 11% of patients at autopsy.[63] They may be multiple in 34% of cases.[63] They are usually incidental findings, most commonly seen in the thoracic spine. The thoracic spine is also the most common level of cord impingement by hemangiomas (Fig. 3–25). Canal compromise by pathologic compression fractures, tumor extension, or hematomas may be seen with hemangiomas. Surgical decompression may be facilitated by preoperative embolization.

Following hemangiomas, giant cell tumors are the most frequent benign neoplasm involving the spinal axis. Similar to metastatic disease, contrast enhancement may more accurately delineate epidural extension of the neoplastic process (Fig. 3–26).

Contrast enhancement may aid in distinguishing pathologic compression fractures by identification of enhancement associated with the neoplastic process.[16] However, partial enhancement may be seen with acute fractures.

VASCULAR RELATED LESIONS

Spinal cord infarctions have an acute onset. Similar to intracranial infarctions, there is initially cord edema, which may be followed by enhancement in the subacute phase. Cord infarcts may be caused by vasculitis, aortic dissections, and postoperative aortic repairs.

Enhancement may also be seen in the more slowly flowing venous channels of cord AVMs (Fig. 3–27). However, contrast usually adds little additional diagnostic information in evaluation of cord AVMs. However, hemosiderin deposition from prior hemorrhage may be differentiated from the slow-flowing venous channels by contrast administration. Cord edema may also be noted.

True cord AVMs present in younger patients, whereas patients with dural fistulas are usually older, with progressive myelopathy. The dilated vessels have a tendency to affect the posterior cord surface.

INFLAMMATORY LESIONS

Epidural abscesses may be identified postoperatively, as previously described. An epidural extension of diskitis or osteomyelitis is usually more reliably defined after contrast administration. Enhancement may be used to follow disease activity, along with resolution of increased signal intensity on T2-weighted sequences.

With the increased use of epidural catheters for pain management by drug infusion, there is an increased need for assessment of those patients who may develop

(Text continues on page 107)

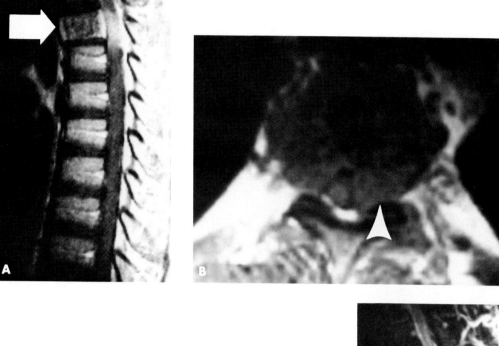

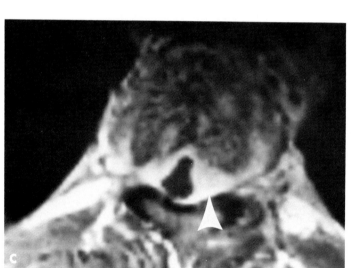

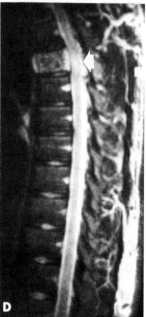

FIGURE 3–25. Hemangioma involving the T-3 vertebral body. **(A)** The sagittal postcontrast (gadopentetate dimeglumine) T1-weighted scan displays the hemangioma (*arrow*), which is markedly enhanced following intravenous administration of contrast material (gadopentetate dimeglumine). The contrast-enhanced scan better defines the epidural component. **(B, C)** Axial pre- and postcontrast scans identify the enhancing epidural component of the hemangioma (*arrowhead*) and the resulting spinal cord compression. **(D)** The sagittal T2-weighted scan reveals the high-signal intensity vertebral body lesion, with both anterior and posterior extension of the tumor. There is also abnormal high-signal intensity with the cord, compatible with edema or gliosis (*arrow*).

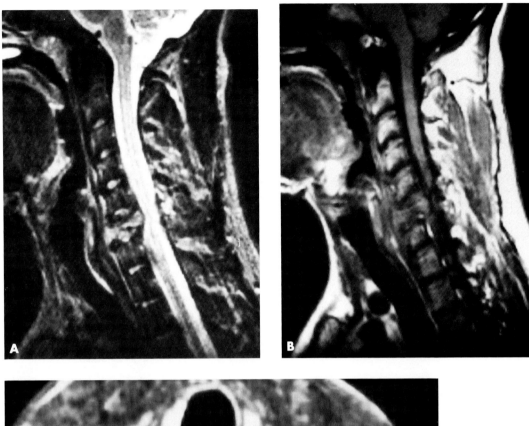

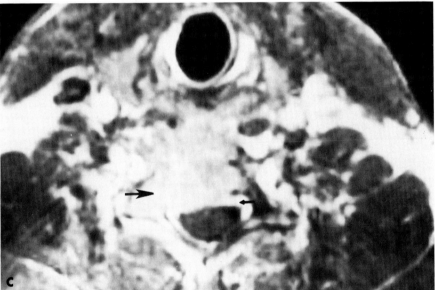

FIGURE 3-26. Giant cell tumor involving the cervical spine. **(A)** The sagittal T2-weighted examination identifies partial compression of the C-6 vertebral body. **(B)** The precontrast T1-weighted examination reveals a soft-tissue mass that encroaches on the ventral subarachnoid space. **(C)** There is marked enhancement of the lesion (*large arrow*) on the postcontrast (gadopentetate dimeglumine) axial T1-weighted scan. Circumferential epidural tumor extension can also be seen postcontrast (*small arrow*).

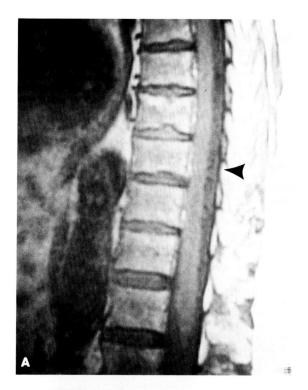

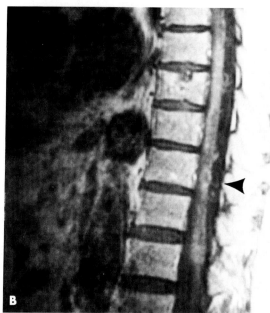

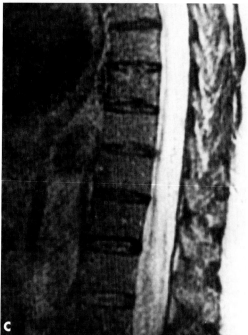

FIGURE 3–27. Lower thoracic cord AVM. **(A)** The T1-weighted sagittal scan faintly identifies the signal flow voids (*arrowhead*) dorsal to the cord. **(B)** Following contrast administration (gadoteridol), the vessels enhance and become slightly more conspicuous. **(C)** The second echo of the T2-weighted series identifies abnormal high-signal intensity within the cord, most likely related to cord edema or gliosis.

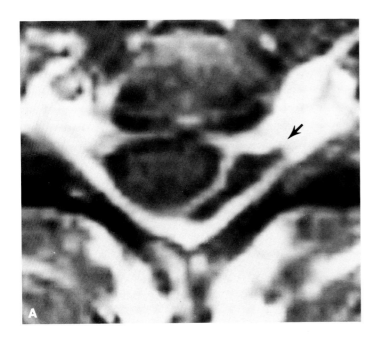

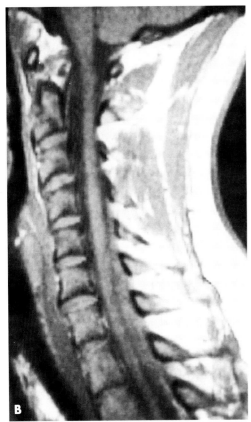

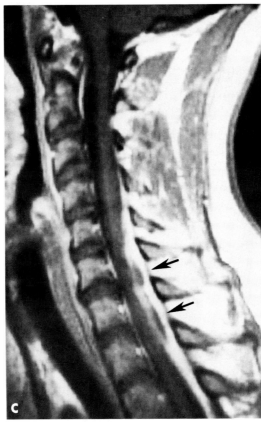

FIGURE 3-28. Surgically verified abscess as a sequela to percutaneous placement of an epidural catheter. **(A)** T1-weighted axial scan after administration of contrast material (gadopentetate dimeglumine). The scan delineates the abscess cavity (*arrow*). **(B, C)** Comparison of the pre- and postcontrast sagittal scans improves delineation of the cavity (*arrows*).

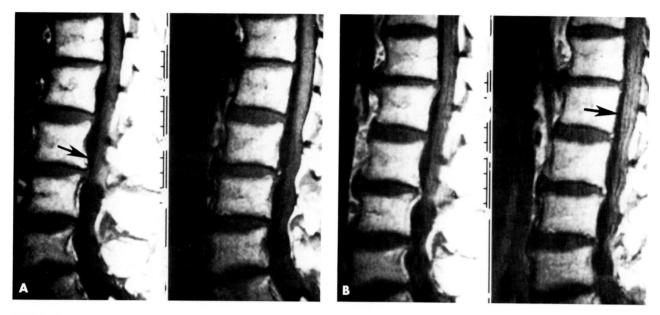

FIGURE 3–29. Arachnoid adhesions from three prior lumbar surgical procedures and several diagnostic myelograms. **(A)** The sagittal precontrast T1-weighted examination identifies clumping of roots (*arrow*). **(B)** Following intravenous administration of contrast material (gadopentetate dimeglumine) there is enhancement of the lumbar roots (*arrow*).

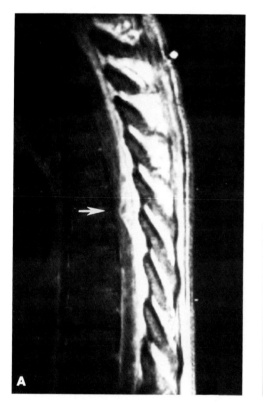

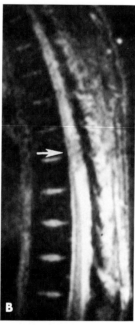

FIGURE 3–30. Disseminated aspergillosis in an immunocompromised patient. There was loculation of the CSF spinal compartment caused by direct involvement of the CSF space. An attempt at a myelogram was unsuccessful. **(A)** The postcontrast (gadopentetate dimeglumine) T1-weighted examination identifies diffuse enhancement of the subarachnoid space and dorsal mass effect upon the cord in the lower thoracic region (*arrow*). **(B)** The T2-weighted scan displays an indistinct abnormal soft-tissue mass in this region, but is less diagnostic than the postcontrast T1-weighted scan.

neurologic symptoms related to the catheter site. Scans following the intravenous administration of contrast material more accurately define the underlying process (i.e., hemorrhage versus inflammatory lesion) (Fig. 3–28).

Arachnoid adhesions caused by prior diagnostic examinations or therapy have displayed various degrees of enhancement, from minimal or nonexistent to moderate, but never striking in degree (Fig. 3–29).[16,57] The role of contrast enhancement for routine diagnosis of arachnoiditis is limited, since in most patients a diagnosis can be made with equal certainty by noncontrast scans.[15] However, cystic cord changes caused by arachnoid adhesions can usually be differentiated from cystic changes or necrosis caused by neoplasia. It may prove possible to distinguish leptomeningeal (tumor) enhancement from arachnoiditis by their different degrees of enhancement.[15]

Meningitis and involvement of the subarachnoid space may be revealed by contrast enhancement in the spine (Fig. 3–30).[64] Loculations and adhesions are possible sequelae. Other reported inflammatory etiologies of cord enhancement include varicella–zoster transverse myelitis.[16] This series, however, reported that most of their cases of transverse myelitis did not enhance. *Transverse myelitis* is defined as an acute pro-

gressive myelopathy without a known neurologic disease. This may be of viral, vasculitic, demyelinating, or postvaccination etiology. Other inflammatory causes of spinal leptomeningeal enhancement include sarcoidosis and chronic shunt therapy.[37]

The central nervous system is involved in 5% to 10% of patients with sarcoidosis. Spinal cord involvement is rare. Intramedullary and pial enhancement are the most frequently encountered patterns. Postradiation myelitis may also demonstrate enhancement.

DEMYELINATING DISEASE

Active areas of involvement of the spinal cord by multiple sclerosis (MS) may enhance. During the active phase there is usually mild cord enlargement or a focal change in contour (Fig. 3–31). Similar to MS in the intracranial compartment, only a few lesions may enhance. At times, differentiation of the plaque from neoplasia may be difficult if a single lesion is present. A concomitant brain MRI may be of benefit to confirm the diagnosis. The true extent of the demyelinating disease usually exceeds the clinical suggestion. The lesions, initially, are larger and ill defined owing to the

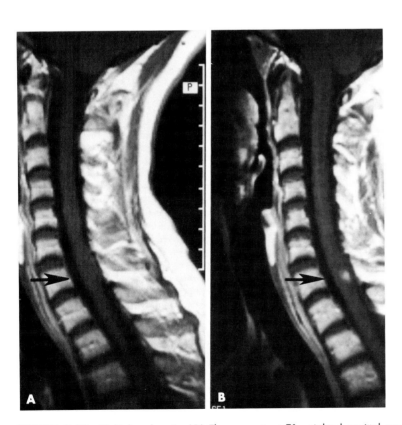
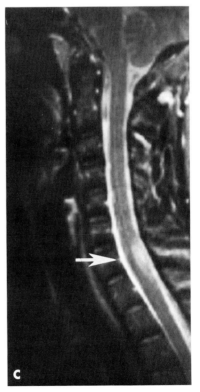

FIGURE 3–31. Multiple sclerosis. **(A)** The precontrast T1-weighted sagittal scan fails to identify the cervical lesion (*arrow*). **(B)** Following contrast administration (gadoteridol) there is enhancement detected in the dorsal aspect of the cord (*arrow*). **(C)** The T2-weighted examination verifies the area of abnormality demonstrated on the contrast-enhanced scan.

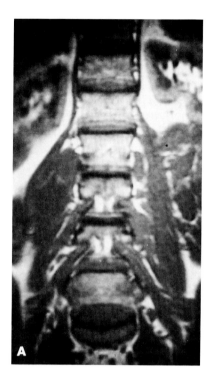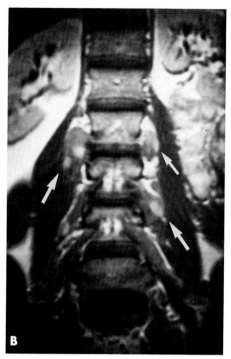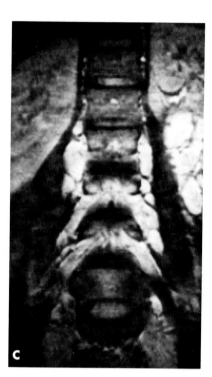

FIGURE 3–32. Multiple, large neurofibromas in the lumbar region (*arrows*). **(A, B)** Pre- and postcontrast (gadoteridol), coronal, T1-weighted scans both identify the paraspinal lesions. Heterogeneous enhancement (*arrows*) is noted postcontrast. **(C)** The coronal, T2-weighted examination readily identifies the masses, which are markedly hyperintense. (Courtesy of Frank W. Morgan, MD)

presence of edema. With time, they become better delineated.[37] They typically have more gliosis than intracranial lesions. Atrophic changes may be seen with extensive involvement. Chronic lesions, typically, do not enhance. Significant numbers of patients will have spinal lesions without intracranial involvement.

Acute disseminated encephalomyelitis (ADEM) may be indistinguishable from MS, with perivascular involvement in the spinal canal. More severe cases may be hemorrhagic. These patients may have a rapidly progressive course.

CONGENITAL LESIONS

Neurofibromatosis is frequently associated with plexiform neurofibromas (Fig. 3–32). There is usually intense enhancement following the intravenous administration of contrast material. These lesions are usually dumbbell-shaped, extending intra- and extradurally, with enlargement of the neuroforamen. Intramedullary tumors may also be seen, such as astrocytomas, ependymomas, central schwannomas, and hamartomas.[65,66]

As previously described, AVMs usually demonstrate enhancement in the slow-flowing venous portions and

variable enhancement of the cord at the involved level.[67] Cavernous hemangiomas may not enhance with contrast administration,[13] similar to intracranial cavernous hemangiomas (Fig. 3–33).

REFERENCES

1. Runge VM. Clinical spin echo imaging. In: Runge VM, ed. Enhanced magnetic resonance imaging. St Louis: CV Mosby, 1989:10–25.
2. Castillo M, Malko JA, Hoffman JC. The bright intervertebral disk: an indirect sign of abnormal spinal bone marrow on T1-weighted MR images. AJNR 1990;11:23–26.
3. Ross JS, Modic MT, Masaryk TJ, et al. Assessment of extradural degenerative disease with Gd-DTPA-enhanced MR imaging: correlation with surgical and pathologic findings. AJNR 1989; 10:1243–1249.
4. Hueftle M, Modic MT, Ross JS, et al. Lumbar spine: postoperative MR imaging with Gd-DTPA. Radiology 1988;167:817–824.
5. Wood ML. Gradient-echo technique. In: Runge VM, ed. Enhanced magnetic resonance imaging. St Louis: CV Mosby, 1989:31–39.
6. Runge VM. Clinical gradient-echo imaging. In: Runge VM, ed. Enhanced magnetic resonance imaging. St Louis: CV Mosby, 1989:40–53.
7. Tsuruda JS, Norman D, Dillon W, et al. Three-dimensional gradient-recalled MR imaging as a screening tool for the diagnosis of cervical radiculopathy. AJNR 1990;10:1263–1271.

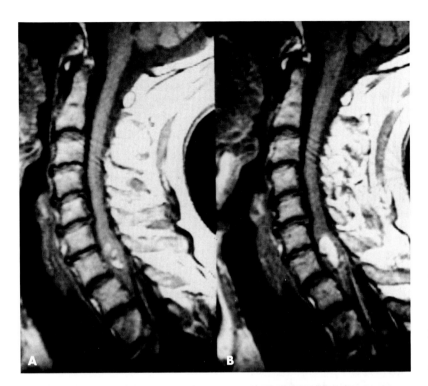

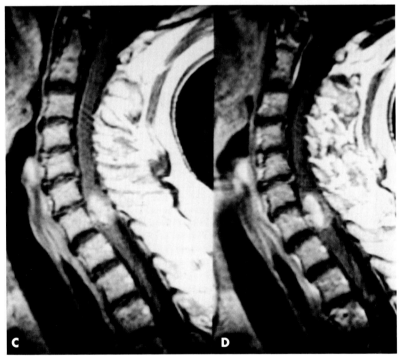

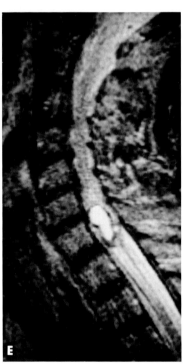

FIGURE 3–33. Cervical spine cavernous hemangioma. **(A, B)** Pre- and **(C, D)** postcontrast (gadoteridol) T1-weighted scans reveal a hemorrhagic lesion with little contrast enhancement. This hemangioma is principally hyperintense on the T2-weighted scan **(E)**, consistent with methemoglobin content. (Courtesy of Steven R. Pollei, MD)

8. Murayama S, Numaguchi Y, Robinson E. The diagnosis of herniated intervertebral disks with MR imaging: a comparison of gradient-refocused-echo and spin-echo pulse sequences. AJNR 1990;11:17–22.

9. VanDyke C, Ross JS, Tkach J, et al. Gradient-echo MR imaging of the cervical spine: evaluation of extradural disease. AJNR 1989;10:627–632.

10. Katz BH, Quencer RM, Hinks RS. Comparison of gradient-recalled-echo and T2-weighted spin-echo pulse sequences in intramedullary spinal lesions. AJNR 1989;10:815–822.

11. Nelson KV, Runge VM. Basic principles. In: Runge VM, ed. Enhanced magnetic resonance imaging. St Louis: CV Mosby, 1989:57–73.

12. Breger RK, Williams AL, Daniels DL, et al. Contrast enhancement in spinal MR imaging. AJNR 1989;10:633–637.

13. Parizel PM, Balériaux D, Rodesch G, et al. Gd-DTPA-enhanced MR imaging of spinal tumors. AJNR 1989;10:249–258.

14. Dillon WP, Norman D, Newton TH, et al. Intradural spinal cord lesions: Gd-DTPA-enhanced MR imaging. Radiology 1989;170:229–237.

15. Johnson CE, Sze G. Benign lumbar arachnoiditis: MR imaging with gadopentetate dimeglumine. AJNR 1990;11:763–770.

16. Sze G, Bravo S, Krol G. Spinal lesions: quantitative and qualitative temporal evolution of gadopentetate dimeglumine enhancement in MR imaging. Radiology 1989;170:849–856.

17. Czervionke LF, Czervionke JM, Daniels DL, Haughton VM. Characteristic features of MR truncation artifacts. AJNR 1988;9:815–824.

18. Yousem DM, Janick PA, Atlas SW, et al. Pseudoatrophy of the cervical portion of the spinal cord on MR images: a manifestation of the truncation artifact. AJNR 1990;11:373–377.

19. Curtin AJ, Chakeres DW, Bulas R, et al. MR imaging artifacts of the axial internal anatomy of the cervical spinal cord. AJNR 1989;10:19–26.

20. Suojanen J, Wang AM, Winston KR. Pantopaque mimicking spinal lipoma: MR pitfall. Case report. J Comput Assist Tomogr 1988;12:346–348.

21. Tsuruda JS, Remley K. Effects of magnetic susceptibility artifacts and motion in evaluating the cervical neural foramina on 3DFT gradient-echo MR imaging. AJNR 1991;12:237–241.

22. Czervionke LF, Daniels DL, Wehrli FW, et al. Magnetic susceptibility artifacts in gradient-recalled echo imaging. AJNR 1988;9:1149–1155.

23. Modic MT. Degenerative disorders of the spine. In: Modic MT, Masaryk TJ, Ross JS, eds. Magnetic resonance imaging of the spine. Chicago: Year Book Medical Publishers, 1989:75–117.

24. Williams MP, Cherryman GB, Husband JR. Significance of thoracic disc herniation demonstrated by MR imaging. J Comput Assist Tomogr 1989;13:211–214.

25. New PFJ, Shoukimas GM. Thoracic spine and spinal cord. In: Stark DD, Bradley WG, eds. Magnetic resonance imaging. St Louis: CV Mosby, 1988:632–665.

26. West JW, Lee C, Dean BL, et al. The role of gadopentetate dimeglumine in the routine evaluation of the lumbar spine. American Roentgen Ray Society annual meeting, 1991 (abstract).

27. Burton CV, Kirkaldy-Willis WH, Young-Hing K, et al. Causes of failure of surgery on the lumbar spine. Clin Orthop 1981;157:191–199.

28. Ross JS, Hueftle MG. Postoperative spine. In Modic MT, Masaryk TJ, Ross JS, eds. Magnetic resonance imaging of the spine. Chicago: Year Book Medical Publishers, 1989:120–148.

29. Sotiropoulos S, Charetz NI, Lang P, et al. Differentiation between postoperative scar and recurrent disk herniation: prospective comparison of MR, CT, and contrast-enhanced CT. AJNR 1989;10:639–643.

30. Ross JS, Masaryk TJ, Schrader M, et al. MR imaging of the postoperative lumbar spine: assessment with gadopentetate dimeglumine. AJNR 1990;11:771–776.

31. Frocrain L, Duvauferrier R, Husson JL, et al. Recurrent postoperative sciatica: evaluation with MR imaging and enhanced CT. Radiology 1989;170:531–533.

32. Ross JS, Modic MT, Masaryk TJ, et al. Assessment of extradural degenerative disease with Gd-DTPA–enhanced MR imaging: correlation with surgical and pathologic findings. AJNR 1989; 10:1243–1249.

33. Coventry MB, Ghormley RK, Kernohan JW. The intervertebral disc: its microscopic anatomy and pathology: III. Changes in the intervertebral disc concomitant with age. J Bone Joint Surg 1945;27.

34. Ross JS, Blaser S, Masaryk TJ, et al. Gd-DTPA enhancement of posterior epidural scar: an experimental model. AJNR 1989;10:1105–1110.

35. Nguyen CM, Ho KC, Yu S, et al. An experimental model to study contrast enhancement in MR imaging of the intervertebral disk. AJNR 1989;10:811–814.

36. Bundschuh CV, Stein L, Slusser JH, et al. Distinguishing between scar and recurrent herniated disk in postoperative patients: value of contrast-enhanced CT and MR imaging. AJNR 1990;11:949–958.

37. Ross JS. Inflammatory disease. In: Modic MT, Masaryk TJ, Ross JS, eds. Magnetic resonance imaging of the spine. Chicago: Year Book Medical Publishers, 1989:167–182.

38. Mirvis SE, Geisler FH, Jelinek JJ, et al. Acute cervical spine trauma: evaluation with 1.5-T MR imaging. Radiology 1988; 166:807–816.

39. Yamashita Y, Takahashi M, Matsuno Y, et al. Chronic injuries of the spinal cord: assessment with MR imaging. Radiology 1990; 175:849–854.

40. Schouman-Claeys E, Frija G, Cuenod CA, et al. MR imaging of acute spinal cord injury: results of an experimental study in dogs. AJNR 1990;11:959–965.

41. Casselman JW, Jolie E, Dehaene I, et al. Gadolinium-enhanced MR imaging of infarction of the anterior spinal cord. Case report. AJNR 1991;11:561.

42. Fetell MR, Stein BM. Spinal tumors. In: Rowland LP, ed. Merritt's textbook of neurology, 8th ed. Philadelphia:Lea & Febiger, 1989.

43. Russell DS, Rubenstein LJ. Pathology of tumors of the nervous system, 5th ed. Baltimore: Williams & Wilkins, 1989.

44. Lim V, Sobel D, Zyroff J. Spinal cord pial metastases: MR imaging with gadopentetate dimeglumine. AJNR 1990;11:975–982.

45. Runge VM, Gelblum DY. The role of gadolinium-diethylenetriaminepentaacetic acid in the evaluation of the central nervous system. Magn Reson Q 1990:6:1–23.

46. Sloof JL, Kernohan JW, MacCarty CS. Primary intramedullary tumors of the spinal cord and filum terminale. Philadelphia: WB Saunders, 1964.

47. Sonneland PR, Scheithauer BW, Onofrio BM. Myxopapillary ependymoma: a clinicopathologic and immunocytochemical study of 77 cases. Cancer 1985;56:883–893.

48. Barone BM, Elvidge AR. Ependymomas: a clinical survey. J Neurosurg 1970;33:428–438.

49. Bydder GM, Brown J, Niendorf HP, Young IR. Enhancement of cervical intraspinal tumors in MR imaging with intravenous gadolinium-DTPA. J Comput Assist Tomogr 1985;9:847–851.

50. Sze G, Krol G, Zimmerman RD, Deck MDF. Intramedullary disease of the spine: diagnosis using gadolinium-DTPA-enhanced MR imaging. AJNR 1988;9:847–858.

51. Cohen AR, Wisoff JH, Allen JC, Epstein F. Malignant astrocytomas of the spinal cord. J Neurosurg 1989;70:50–54.

52. Berns DH, Blaser S, Ross JS, et al. MR imaging with Gd-DTPA in leptomeningeal spread of lymphoma. J Comput Assist Tomogr 1988;12:499–500.

53. Sze G, Abramson A, Krol G, et al. Gadolinium-DTPA in the evaluation of intradural extramedullary spinal disease. AJNR 1988;9:153–163.

54. Sze G. Gadolinium-DTPA in spinal disease. Radiol Clin North Am 1988;26:1009–1024.

55. Gautier-Smith PC. Clinical aspects of spinal neurofibromas. Brain 1967;90:359–393.

56. Dorwart RH, Wara WM, Norman D, Levin VA. Complete myelographic evaluation of spinal metastases from medulloblastoma. Radiology 1981;139:403–408.

57. Sze G, Krol G, Zimmerman RD, Deck MD. Malignant extradural spinal tumors: MR imaging with Gd-DTPA. Radiology 1988;167:217–223.

58. Sze G, Stimac GK, Bartlet C, et al. Multicenter study of gadopentetate dimeglumine as an MR contrast agent: evaluation in patients with spinal tumors. AJNR 1990;11:967–974.

59. Avrahami E, Tadmor R, Dally O, Hadar H. Early MR demonstration of spinal metastases in patients with normal radiographs and CT and radionuclide bone scans. J Comput Assist Tomogr 1989;13:598–602.

60. Gilbert RW, Kim J, Posner JB. Epidural spinal cord compression from metastatic tumor: diagnosis and treatment. Ann Neurol 1978;3:40–51.

61. Stimac G, Porter B, Olson D, et al. Gadolinium-DTPA-enhanced MR imaging of spinal neoplasms: preliminary investigation and comparison with unenhanced spin-echo and STIR sequences. AJNR 1988;9:839–846.

62. Schmorl G, Junghanns H. The human spine in health and disease, 2nd ed. New York: Grune & Stratton, 1971.

63. Osborn RE, Mojtahedi S. CT myelography of cauda equina actinomycosis. J Comput Assist Tomogr 1987;11:361–362.

64. Burk DL, Brunberg JA, Kanal E, et al. Spinal and paraspinal neurofibromatosis: surface coil MR imaging at 1.5 T. Radiology 1987;162:797–801.

65. Lewis TT, Kingsley DPE. Magnetic resonance imaging of multiple spinal neurofibromata–neurofibromatosis. Neuroradiology 1987;29:562–564.

66. Terwey B, Becker H, Thron AK, Vahldiek G. Gadolinium-DTPA enhanced MR imaging of spinal dural arteriovenous fistulas. J Comput Assist Tomogr 1989;13:30–37.

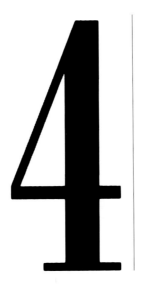

Application of Magnetic Resonance Contrast Agents in Body Imaging

Graeme M. Bydder

Progress in the clinical use of contrast agents has been faster in the central nervous system (CNS) than it has been elsewhere in the body. Intravenous gadopentetate dimeglumine (Gd-DTPA) is now widely accepted as a contrast agent of proved value in diseases of the CNS, but there is less certainty about its role for applications elsewhere in the body. The blood–brain barrier very largely confines this agent to an intravascular distribution in normal circumstances and creates a valuable role for it as a marker of disease when this barrier is disrupted. These favorable circumstances do not prevail elsewhere in the body, where the distribution of gadopentetate dimeglumine is a much more dynamic process, and precise timing and dosage is more critical in determining its effectiveness.

In spite of these difficulties, there is wide scope for the use of contrast agents in the body. The increased availability of subsecond-imaging techniques means that dynamic magnetic resonance imaging (MRI) is now a realistic possibility in many situations. The clinical use of reticuloendothelial agents has just begun, and the liver provides options for the imaginative application of MR chemistry. In keeping with the overall intention of this volume, emphasis will be placed on the clinical results and applications that are now achievable. The material in this chapter has also been the subject of several recent reviews.[1–3]

AVAILABLE CONTRAST AGENTS

Although a large number of parenteral agents are in the developmental stage, only gadopentetate dimeglumine is routinely available for clinical use, and emphasis is placed on the use of this agent.

Intravenous magnetic iron oxide particles (MIOPs) show considerable promise as reticuloendothelial agents, but three of the first 99 patients studied experienced hypotensive episodes, and new formulations of MIOPs are being developed. These are undergoing early clinical trials, but are not yet available for general use.

A wide variety of oral agents are available for labeling the gut as an important component of the MRI examination of the abdomen and pelvis, but the most important two agents are oral gadopentetate dimeglumine and MIOPs. There have been some difficulties in formulating gadopentetate dimeglumine for oral use. Furthermore, although Phase III trials have been undertaken for bowel labeling with MIOPs, this agent is not yet available for general use.

TECHNIQUES

It is very important to use MR contrast agents with the appropriate imaging technique. One of the early observations following introduction of intravenous gadopentetate dimeglumine was that highly T1-weighted sequences displayed contrast enhancement in situations for which heavily T2-weighted sequences did not. The basis for this is well understood. Paramagnetic agents decrease both T1 and T2. The decrease in T1 tends to increase signal intensity with most commonly used pulse sequences, whereas the decrease in T2 tends to decrease signal intensity. With low concentrations of gadopentetate dimeglumine, the first effect is dominant, but with high concentrations the second effect becomes more important, so that the two effects may cancel out, producing no net change,

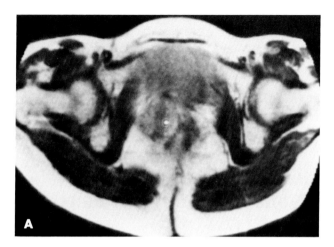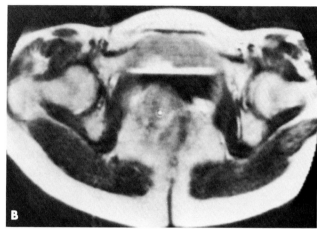

FIGURE 4-1 Patient with a pelvic tumor. T1-weighted spin echo images before **(A)** and after **(B)** intravenous gadopentetate dimeglumine administration. Following enhancement **(B)** the urine anteriorly in the bladder is unchanged. Below this there is an area of increased signal where the T1-shortening effects of gadopentetate dimeglumine are dominant. Posteriorly, where the concentration of the contrast agent is high, there is a reduction in signal intensity from T2 shortening.

or even a loss, of signal intensity. In most organs, with the usual range of gadopentetate dimeglumine doses, the increase in signal intensity is all that is usually observed, but in urine in which this agent is concentrated and the T1 and T2 are long, a loss of signal intensity is frequently observed (Fig. 4–1).

The net effect depends not only on the dose of gadopentetate dimeglumine, but on its distribution, the timing postcontrast, the choice of pulse sequences for the examination, and the operating field strength, as well as the initial T1 and T2 of both the normal and abnormal tissues that are under study. In assessing the net benefit of the contrast agent, it is strictly necessary to take all of these factors into account, and some of the variation in results reflects a choice of different options among these factors.

Systematic assessment of the effect of some of these variables has been carried out in studies of the CNS and, to a lesser extent, in the rest of the body. Many of the effects can reasonably be inferred from a knowledge of the distribution of metallic chelates used in nuclear medicine and from experience with iodinated contrast agents used in x-ray computed tomography (CT), but a major difference is the effect of pulse sequences. The importance of using T1-weighted sequences has already been noted, but there are several other choices of imaging techniques that can have a major impact on the observed enhancement.

Sequences employing gradient-recalled echoes have achieved increasing popularity over the last 3 years. They consist of a radiofrequency (rf) pulse (classically of 90°, but often reduced below this or increased beyond it), followed by a conventional data acquisition without an intervening 180° pulse. When the rf pulse is low (10° to 30°) the T1 weighting is usually small, but if the angle is increased to 110° to 135°, T1 weighting is often increased. The T2 weighting increases with the echo time (TE). In comparison with spin echo sequences, the lack of a 180° pulse means that the sequence is more sensitive to susceptibility effects and displays phase-dependent chemical shift effects. When the radiofrequency pulse angle is low, much of the magnetization is stored in the long axis; consequently, it is possible to achieve fast imaging with a relatively good signal-to-noise ratio. This has been important in performing dynamic studies and in volume acquisitions for which a great deal of data are acquired in a relatively short time. In spite of having only a moderate T1 dependence, gradient-recalled echoes, with a reduced flip angle, have been used for dynamic studies with reasonable success.

More recently, the repetition time (TR) has been further shortened with certain types of gradient echo sequences, such that images can be acquired within 0.5 to 1 second. This very fast imaging allows acquisition in a dynamic mode and is important in body studies, which may otherwise be compromised by the presence of respiratory or peristaltic motion. To ensure that the sequence has a strong T1 dependence, a prepatory 180°-inverting pulse is applied. The period of longitudinal recovery before the rf pulse allows variable recovery and may be used to provide highly T1-dependent contrast.

An even more rapid approach to image acquisition

is provided by echo planar imaging (EPI), for which the whole data collection is performed in periods of about 20 to 100 ms. This technique requires strong gradients, and the signal-to-noise ratio can be low. In spite of this, impressive 128 × 128 matrix images of the abdomen have been obtained without significant motion artifact. The cycle can be repeated every 1 to 2 seconds to allow time for the longitudinal magnetization to recover. The standard EPI images are T2 weighted, but, as with very fast gradient-recalled images, an 180°-inverting pulse can be used to increase the sensitivity of the sequence to changes in T1.

Both the fast gradient-recalled approach and EPI have an increased sensitivity to susceptibility effects and, therefore, are particularly sensitive to the effects of MIOPs.

Another class of pulse sequences of importance in body applications are those involving fat suppression.[4] Fat has a short T1, and enhancement with gadopentetate dimeglumine may reduce the T1 of a tissue of interest into the fat range, with a resultant loss of conspicuity with fatty tissues. The wide distribution of fat and its presence at tissue planes means that this can lead to problems in interpretation in disease outside of the CNS. Several techniques have been developed for effectively suppressing the signal from fat. These involve frequency-selective pulses, either for the fat or water resonance, followed by a dephasing pulse (in the case of fat). These pulses are particularly sensitive to field inhomogeneity. They are relatively easy to implement in areas of the body with small cross sections, such as the neck. There are more difficulties in areas of the body with large cross sections, such as the pelvis. Work is progressing in this area, and a combination of approaches of frequency-selective, binomial pulses and phase-sensitive sequences may be best.

There has also been renewed interest in rapid methods of spin echo imaging, combining some features of EPI with conventional imaging. These may allow examination of the liver in breathholding times with a consequent reduction in motion artifact.[5]

APPLICATION IN CLINICAL PRACTICE

Bronchogenic Carcinoma

One of the advantages of MR over CT in imaging the mediastinum and pulmonary hilum that was recognized early on was that a contrast agent is unnecessary to identify blood vessels and distinguish these from other structures within the mediastinum and hila of the lung. Conventional spin echo sequences usually produce a low-signal intensity from rapidly flowing blood as a re-

sult of dephasing effects. With appropriate selection of the imaging plane, this loss of signal intensity can be so distinct that vessels are readily distinguished from soft-tissue masses.

Although the spatial resolution of MRI is inferior to CT, its soft-tissue contrast is frequently greater, so that the end result in several studies has been a rough equivalence between the results of CT and MRI in clinical problems such as the staging of bronchogenic carcinoma, for which both techniques have the potential to contribute significant clinical information. The problems with both techniques arise because abnormal nodes are recognized only by an increase in size. Unfortunately, some nodes that are not enlarged may contain tumor, and some enlarged nodes may demonstrate reactive changes, but do not contain tumor.

As a consequence of these difficulties, it was concluded by Glazer and associates that accurate staging of the pulmonary hilum was not possible by MRI or CT in patients with lung cancer.[6] In a study of 85 patients with lung cancer, Grenier and co-workers also concluded that both MRI and CT displayed poor sensitivity and marginal specificity for detection of nodal metastases and chest wall involvement.[7] Similar results have been reported by the Radiologic Diagnostic Oncology Group.[8] There has been little indication that contrast agents can improve this situation. It is possible that mediastinal lymphography may improve the results of diagnosis with MRI and CT, but contrast agents to perform these techniques are not yet available.

Myocardial Infarction

Gated MRI has been used for identifying and quantifying myocardial infarction, and there has been considerable interest in the possibility that gadopentetate dimeglumine may improve the accuracy of MRI in diagnosing the extent of myocardial infarction.

Although T2-weighted images are reasonably accurate in depicting myocardial infarction, there are potential pitfalls because adjacent slow-flowing blood may also produce a high-signal intensity. There may also be difficulties in interpretation owing to residual motion artifact.

Gadopentetate dimeglumine has been used for detection of acute myocardial infarction in dogs, with the T1 from the infarcted area postcontrast being shorter than that from the normal area. In acutely damaged myocardium, gadopentetate dimeglumine may accumulate in the infarcted area as a result of collateral circulation, revascularization, and cellular damage, all of which may reduce washout from the affected zone. By 10 to 15 minutes, much of this agent is lost from the normal tissue, but it may persist in the zone of injury. Contrast enhancement may typically be seen during the first 2 weeks after acute infarction, but it is not seen in the chronic phase after myocardial scar has been formed.[9-12]

De Roos and colleagues have described four different patterns of enhancement:[11-13]

1. Uniform diffuse enhancement
2. Predominant subendocardial enhancement
3. Inhomogeneous enhancement, with dark areas in or adjacent to enhanced infarct, possibly as a result of hemorrhage or differences in the degree of edema or collateral circulation
4. A doughnut pattern with a nonenhancing core, which may be due to a central zone of no reflow

Similar enhancement patterns were observed in both reperfused and nonreperfused infarcts.

There are indications that MRI performed early after administration of gadopentetate dimeglumine is capable of differentiating reperfused from nonreperfused infarcts after treatment with fibrinolysis. It may also be possible to demonstrate a reduction in apparent infarct size with successful reperfusion.

Techniques for estimating cardiac size, based on the use of intravenous gadopentetate dimeglumine have been implemented by de Roos and associates[14] (Fig. 4–2). When combined with subsecond imaging, gado-

pentetate dimeglumine may provide an assessment of myocardial perfusion[15] that could be of clinical value.

Breast

General results of enhancement in about 1000 MR studies of the breast with gadopentetate dimeglumine, performed by Heywang and co-workers,[16,17] indicate that

- All carcinomas enhance significantly.
- Focal enhancement may also occur in fibroadenomas, papillomas, and some cases of focal proliferative dysplasia.
- Diffuse enhancement is most frequently encountered in proliferative dysplasia or within inflammatory changes and, less frequently, in cases of malignancy.
- No significant enhancement is noted in nonproliferative dysplasia, normal breast, old scarring, and cysts.
- Evaluation of the speed of enhancement shows a fast rise in signal intensity in most carcinomas and a delayed rise in many benign lesions, but delayed enhancement cannot be used as a reliable criterion for the exclusion of malignancy, since a few carcinomas show delayed enhancement.

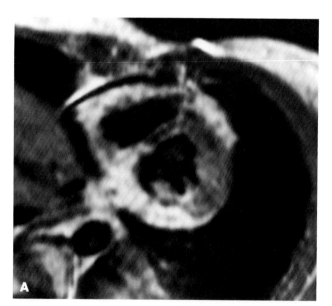 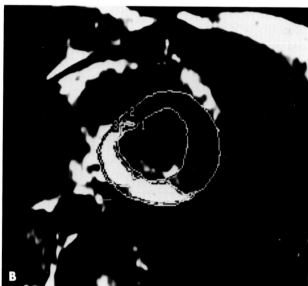

FIGURE 4-2 Short axis view of enhancement of an inferior wall myocardial infarction following intravenous gadopentetate dimeglumine administration **(A)**. The infarct size can be estimated by tracing the area of enhancement **(B)** and expressing it as a percentage of the cross-sectional area on serial sections. (Courtesy of Dr. Albert de Roos, University Hospital, Leiden, The Netherlands)

From these results, Heywang has proposed the following rules for image interpretation:

1. In cases in which there is no significant enhancement, malignancy larger than the slice thickness can be excluded.
2. If focal enhancement is present, further investigation (biopsy) is usually necessary to distinguish malignancy, benign tumors, and rarely, focal proliferative dysplasia.
3. Diffuse enhancement is very nonspecific. A biopsy is recommended if there is any suggestion that a focal abnormality exists.

The most useful result of these studies is the high negative predictive value that the absence of contrast enhancement has for the exclusion of malignancy. The technique is of value in differentiating irregular dysplasia and carcinoma, differentiating between carcinoma and scar (provided that at least 6 months have elapsed since surgery or 18 months since radiotherapy), and evaluating radiographically dense breasts (to detect or determine the extent of malignancy) where there is high clinical suspicion. This includes situations in which there is probably a palpable abnormality, a primary tumor is being sought, further malignancy is being excluded, or limited surgery is planned for a small carcinoma. A case in whom mammography was unhelpful, but intravenous gadopentetate dimeglumine displayed marked enhancement, is seen in Figure 4–3.

Liver and Spleen

In the first studies of liver metastases with intravenous gadopentetate dimeglumine, using highly T1-weighted sequences, the difference in signal intensity between the lesions and normal liver was reduced following contrast administration. This was attributed to accumulation of the drug in the extracellular compartment. This space is relatively small in the normal liver, but is considerably enlarged in metastases. During the long data acquisitions (several minutes) used in early studies, gadopentetate dimeglumine diffused into the lesions, which tended to become isointense with surrounding normal liver.[18] However, with T1-weighted spin echo or partial saturation sequences, administration of this agent did reveal some tumors that otherwise were poorly demonstrated (Fig. 4–4). Some metastases also became more obvious as a result of their lack of enhancement (Fig. 4–5).

Faster-imaging techniques make it possible to acquire data immediately after bolus administration of gadopentetate dimeglumine so that differences in signal intensity between hypervascular lesions and normal liver can be increased (when images are acquired within the first 2 to 3 minutes postcontrast). Clinical studies have shown that hypervascular metastases demonstrate greater enhancement than normal liver in the first few minutes. A decrease in signal intensity then occurs after about a further minute, and the lesion typically became isointense 5 to 10 minutes after contrast injection. The enhancement is generally inhomogeneous.[19–21]

Hepatocellular carcinomas may show a hypervascular or hypovascular pattern. Like metastases the pattern of enhancement is usually inhomogeneous. In 75% of the cases, hepatocellular carcinoma showed no areas of high-signal intensity in the late phase of the examination, but in 43%, a peripheral halo, with delayed enhancement in the area of the pseudocapsule, was observed.[22]

Hemangiomas typically show a marked increase in signal intensity; accordingly, they are visualized as hyperintense lesions in the late phase. The fill-in phenomenon may be very obvious, but this is not invariable.[21–22]

Yoshida and colleagues compared the contrast-enhancement patterns in 22 patients with hepatocellular carcinoma and in 18 patients with hemangiomas.[22] With hepatocellular carcinoma, there was a hyperintense mass before contrast enhancement in 32%, peak enhancement occurred at about 10 seconds after injection in 55%, slight to moderate peak enhancement was seen in 73%, there was absent or minimally delayed enhancement in 100%, and a capsule or nodular appearance was present in 59%. With hemangioma there was a hypointense mass before enhancement in 72%, peak enhancement occurred more than 2 minutes after injection in 72%, there was marked peak enhancement in 83%, and moderate to marked delayed enhancement in 100%.

In another study, Hamm and associates investigated the appearance of metastases and hemangiomas using conventional T1- and T2-weighted sequences, as well as delayed post contrast (11 and 60 minutes) MRI.[21] In dynamic studies, hemangiomas were characterized by peripheral contrast enhancement, with subsequent fill-in (enhancement) of the initially hypointense lesion center. Metastases showed very mixed patterns of enhancement, and their signal intensity remained low compared with that of liver. In delayed postcontrast examinations, some hemangiomas had a very high and homogeneous signal intensity, whereas metastases were characterized by inhomogeneous and hyperintense to isointense signal intensity. The contrast between tumor and liver was higher in all hemangiomas than it was for metastases. Focal nodular hyperplasia typically shows immediate enhancement, reaching a maximum within the first minute postcontrast, followed by a decrease in signal intensity.

(Text continues on page 120)

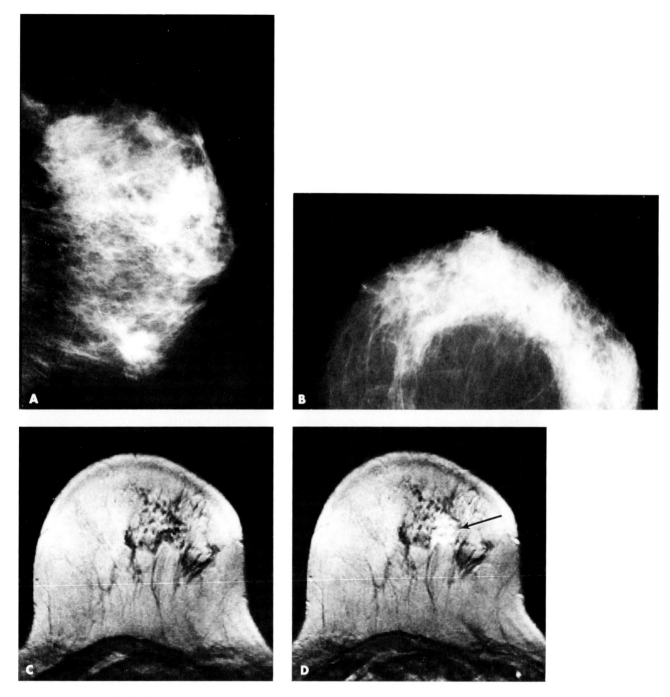

FIGURE 4-3 Nonpalpable breast cancer. Dense breast on mammography, with mass lesion on MRI demonstrating marked enhancement. Mammography-mediolateral **(A)** and craniocaudal **(B)** views; MR images before **(C)** and after **(D)** intravenous gadopentetate dimeglumine. The tumor *(arrow)* is well seen postcontrast owing to its enhancement. (Courtesy of Dr. S.H. Heywang-Kobrunner, Radiol Klink und Poliklinik Klinikum Grossharden, Munich FRG)

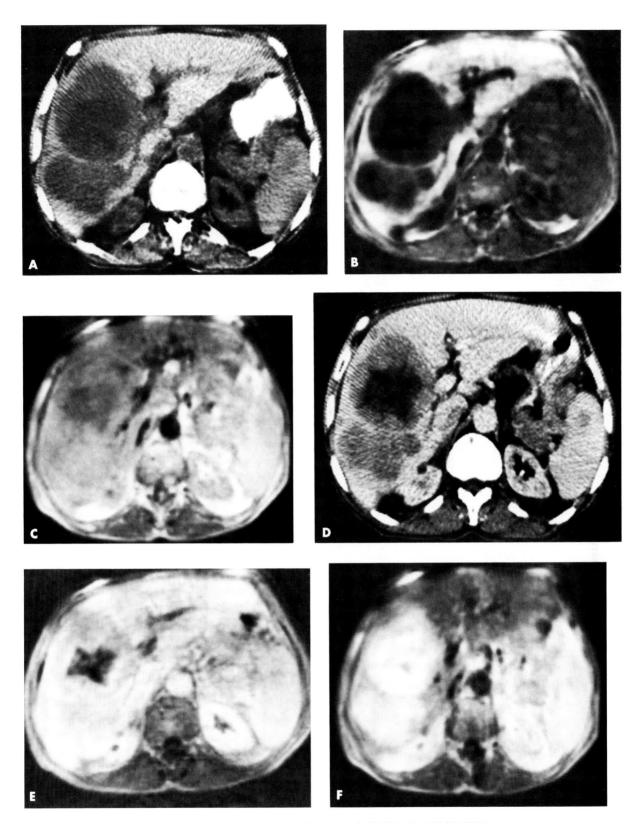

FIGURE 4-4 Multiple metastases: sequence comparison. Unenhanced CT **(A)**, IR1400/13/400 **(B)**, and PS1000/13 **(C)** images compared with **(D)** postcontrast CT, and post-gadopentetate dimeglumine MRI, with the same **(E)** inversion recovery and **(F)** partial saturation techniques. Although much of the largest tumor becomes isointense following enhancement in **E**, the metastases are highlighted in **F**.

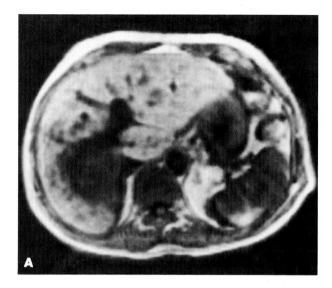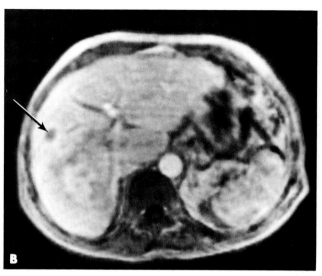

FIGURE 4-5 Liver metastases. Inversion recovery images before **(A)** and after **(B)** intravenous gadopentetate dimeglumine. Although the larger metastasis is less obvious in **B**, a smaller metastasis is more obvious postcontrast *(arrow)*.

Magnetic resonance arterial portography has also been performed and has been of value in increasing lesion conspicuity.[23]

Magnetic iron oxide particles have been used in a few clinical trials.[24–26] They are injected intravenously and subsequently lodge in the reticuloendothelial system. The particles are characteristically superparamagnetic in that a normal applied magnetic field produces a relatively strong induced field that disappears when the applied field is removed. The effect of these particles is to introduce microscopic inhomogeneities into the tissues, such that rapid dephasing occurs and there is a drastic reduction in the tissue T2 (or T2*). The iron dose required is about 1 mg/kg, which is similar to the absolute dose for oral iron replacement therapy. The iron subsequently enters the body iron stores.

Initial clinical trials demonstrated acute toxicity in the form of hypotension in 3 of 99 cases. The mechanism of this adverse effect is not understood, and intense study is under way to develop safe formulations and strategies for clinical use.

Gradient echo and echo planar imaging show increased sensitivity to the effects of MIOPs, allowing a two- to fourfold reduction in dose.

Manganese DPDP shows promise as a hepatobiliary contrast agent that generally increases the tumor–liver contrast-to-noise ratio and improves visualization of focal lesions.[27, 28]

Dynamic MR studies of focal lesions in the spleen using gadopentetate dimeglumine have demonstrated greater lesion conspicuity than conventional T1- and T2-weighted imaging.[29]

Bowel Labeling

The need for a bowel-labeling agent has been obvious since the first studies with abdominal MRI. Numerous agents have been proposed, and many have been tried in healthy volunteers and patients. Positive agents increase intraluminal signal intensity compared with normal bowel contents. These include oils and fats, as well as paramagnetic agents such as iron salts and gadopentetate dimeglumine.

Gas-providing substances, perfluorocarbons (PFCs), and MIOPs act as negative agents. Gas has a very low proton density, and PFCs are compounds in which protons are replaced by fluorine atoms.[30] The MIOPs selectively decrease T2.

Formulation of gadopentetate dimeglumine in a concentration of 1 mmol/L, with the addition of mannitol at 15 g/L, gives satisfactory filling of the bowel.[31]

Magnetic iron particles with a diameter of 3.5 μm, containing Fe_2O_3 and Fe_3O_4, have been produced with a polymer coating. A viscous solution is preferred to an aqueous one.[32–34]

Positive agents increase the artifacts seen on MR images caused by bowel motion. However, moving structures with a very low signal intensity, such as that provided by opacification of the bowel with negative-contrast agents, produce little artifact.

Minimal side effects have been reported with both gadopentetate dimeglumine and MIOPs. Current issues include assessment of the extent to which MIOPs obliterate signal from organs and lesions adjacent to bowel. There are also difficulties in obtaining full opacification of both small and large bowel.

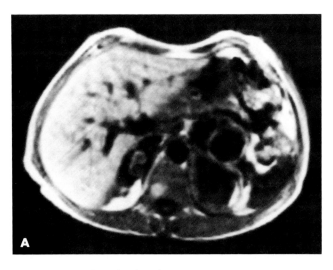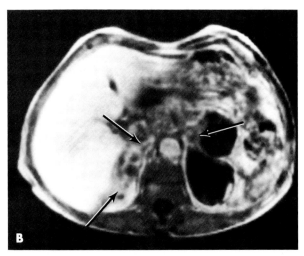

FIGURE 4-6 Bilateral adrenal metastases. Inversion recovery images before **(A)** and after **(B)** intravenous gadopentetate dimeglumine. Mild enhancement is seen within neoplastic tissue *(arrows)* permitting solid tumor to be differentiated from cysts.

Kidney

There are several issues concerning the kidney. One is the effectiveness of contrast agents in diagnosis of structural lesions and another is the effectiveness of contrast agents in assessing the functional status of the kidney.

The advent of faster gradient echo techniques with reduced flip angles has permitted a better approach to assessing the functional status of the kidney.[35–38] Depending on arterial blood flow, an increase in signal intensity can be observed 10 to 20 seconds after bolus injection of intravenous gadopentetate dimeglumine (0.1 mmol/kg). A maximum value is reached 20 to 50 seconds after the first signs of enhancement, followed by a constant slow fall in signal intensity. The T1 reduction produced by gadopentetate dimeglumine provides an early increase in signal intensity in the renal cortex. Ultrafiltration and dilution in the extravascular space produces the subsequent slow decrease. In the medulla, an increase in signal intensity can be observed 10 to 20 seconds later than in the cortex. The signal intensity decreases 30 to 40 seconds after the first sign of enhancement.

Retention of water results in concentration of gadopentetate dimeglumine in the collecting ducts and urine. The contrast agent then passes into the calyces, with the T2-shortening effects of the agent dominating (owing to the increased concentration of contrast agent) and producing a loss of signal intensity.

Renal masses may display precontrast signal intensity similar to that of the surrounding normal tissue; therefore, anatomic deformation of some type is necessary for diagnosis. The definition of lesions is improved with gadopentetate dimeglumine. Few renal lesions display early enhancement; most show reduced and delayed enhancement or no enhancement. Results may be improved by the use of fat-saturation techniques with contrast enhancement.[39] Contrast administration is also of value in demonstrating retroperitoneal extrarenal masses, which may displace or compress the kidneys.

Dynamic studies can be performed by plotting signal intensity values in the renal cortex and medulla against time. In acute obstruction of the urinary tract, enhancement of the renal cortex that is observed on dynamic MRI is similar to that in normal patients. The enhancement of renal medulla, however, is greater than normal. The ductal and excretory phases of enhancement are delayed. In chronic obstruction, cortical enhancement is less than normal, with the ductal phase of contrast enhancement diminished or absent. Good correlation has been obtained between contrast-enhanced MRI and iodine-131 hippurate nuclear medicine studies.[37]

Adrenal Glands

Adrenal masses are relatively common. Most of these are normally inactive adenomas, but the adrenal glands are also a preferred site for spread of blood-borne metastases, and MRI has been reasonably successful in differential diagnosis.[40–42] Enhancement of adrenal masses is readily demonstrated postcontrast (Fig. 4–6), with dynamic techniques favored for differential diagnosis.[43] Following bolus injection, enhancement of the adrenal gland is seen within the first minute, with a maximum after 2 to 3 minutes, followed by a reduction in signal intensity as the contrast agent is washed out. Adenomas display only moderate enhancement, whereas malignant lesions display a more distinct increase in signal intensity, followed by a slower washout. The increased signal intensity may persist for 10 to 15 minutes. By using unenhanced images with T2 weighting, overall accuracy in diagnosis is about 70% to 75%. Contrast-enhanced gradient echo sequences may help in the equivocal cases, and a definitive diagnosis can be established in about 90%.

Pelvis

Magnetic resonance imaging can be used as a primary imaging modality for staging of endometrial, cervical, and vaginal carcinoma.[44] Gadopentetate dimeglumine improves tissue differentiation.

In the past, T2-weighted images have been advocated to demonstrate zonal anatomy, but this can also be shown with T1-weighted images postcontrast. The mucosa and endometrium enhance, whereas the junctional zone remains of lower-signal intensity owing to its reduced extracellular space. The paracervical tissue and inner mucosal surface demonstrate enhancement, whereas the cervical tissue remains of low intensity. The mucus of the vagina shows marked enhancement with a low-signal intensity central region. The ovaries also show enhancement, except for cysts. In leiomyoma of the uterus, gadopentetate dimeglumine enhancement demonstrates two patterns: nondegenerate leiomyomas do not usually enhance following IV contrast administration, whereas degenerate and vascular leiomyomas demonstrate varying degrees of enhancement.[45–47]

After intravenous gadopentetate dimeglumine administration, endometrial carcinoma demonstrates enhancement similar to that of myometrium, but less than that of the endometrium. Gadopentetate dimeglumine helps in differentiating viable tumor from necrosis or residual secretions in the endometrial canal. In studies to date, the use of this agent has not significantly improved the assessment of tumor invasion. In the future, fat-saturation techniques, employed with contrast enhancement, may prove valuable here.

Clinical staging of cervical carcinoma may be inaccurate for involvement of the parametrium, pelvic side wall, paraaortic nodes, and the degree of involvement of the uterine body. With T2-weighted images, cervical cancer usually has a high-signal intensity that can be distinguished from the normally low-signal intensity cervical stroma. T1-weighted images provide good differentiation between cervical tumor and pelvic tissue. Overall, the use of gadopentetate dimeglumine does not increase diagnostic accuracy, but tumor heterogeneity is better demonstrated following contrast administration (Fig. 4–7).

Enhancement of primary bladder tumors increases the contrast between bladder wall and associated blood clot on T1-weighted sequences. However, the contrast between fat and perivesical tumor extension, lymph nodes, and bone metastases is usually reduced.[48,49] The signal intensity from the bladder is variable postcontrast and depends on the length of the examination, as well as the patient's renal function. Layering is frequently observed with gadopentetate dimeglumine. Flow effects may be seen, especially in relation to the ureteric orifices.

Enhancement of primary tumors is usually heterogeneous and unrelated to their histology. Intravesical clot does not enhance, and this may be useful for distinguishing it from adjacent tumor. Recurrent and residual tumor usually increases in signal intensity with T1-weighted images following intravenous gadopentetate dimeglumine administration. However, both normal and abnormal bladder wall (and surrounding structures) may also demonstrate an increase in signal intensity postcontrast. Enhancement of the mucosa may occur after instrumentation, radiotherapy, or chemotherapy. Enhancement of the bladder wall has been observed up to 4 years after radiation therapy.

Musculoskeletal Tumors

Generally, T1- and T2-weighted spin echo images are used to stage musculoskeletal tumors. To some extent, heterogeneity favors malignancy, whereas a more uniform pattern may be seen with benign tumors. Extensive edema is usually a sign of malignant tumor.

As with other areas of the body, gadopentetate dimeglumine may be of value in distinguishing viable from necrotic tissue (Fig. 4–8). Most malignant tumors exhibit a rapid increase in signal intensity after bolus contrast injection. The pattern of uptake with benign tumors is slower. This may be a useful sign for differentiating tumors; however, necrotic malignant tumors also show a slower uptake. This can also be found following radiation therapy.[50, 51] On the other hand, some benign aggressive giant cell tumors may show rapid uptake. Following treatment, uptake is generally reduced in responders, but less for nonresponders. Gadopentetate dimeglumine may also be of considerable value in identifying tumor recurrence.

CONCLUSION

For practical purposes the only parenteral agent that is now available for clinical use is gadopentetate dimeglumine, although this compound will be followed by other gadolinium chelates in the near future. These are likely to have similar relaxation properties. Intra-

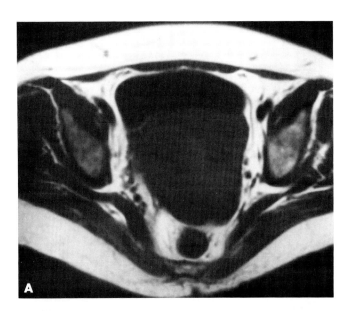

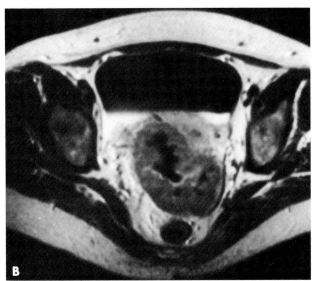

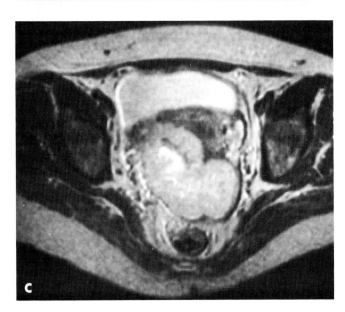

FIGURE 4-7 Fallopian tube carcinoma. Axial T1-weighted spin-echo images before **(A)** and after **(B)** intravenous gadopentetate dimeglumine, compared with **(C)** a T2-weighted (TR/TE = 2000/60) image. The heterogeneity of the tumor is best seen following enhancement **(B)**. (Courtesy of Dr. Hedvig Hricak, University of California, San Francisco)

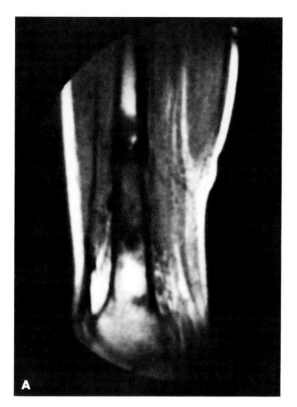
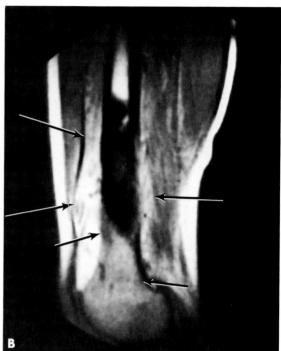

FIGURE 4-8 Osteosarcoma. Inversion recovery images before **(A)** and after **(B)** intravenous gadopentetate dimeglumine administration. Following enhancement, areas within bone *(short arrows)* as well as in the surrounding involved soft tissue show enhancement *(long arrows)*.

venous magnetic iron oxide particles (MIOPs), although very effective, are likely to require a further period of evaluation over several years before fears about their possible toxicity can be allayed.

Both gadopentetate dimeglumine and MIOPs can be used as bowel-labeling agents, without the same concerns about toxicity. Other paramagnetic agents may also prove to be useful for opacification of the gastrointestinal tract.

The use of faster-imaging techniques using gradient-recalled pulse sequences and echo planar imaging has made dynamic imaging possible. Fat-suppression techniques may also be of considerable value in the body in avoiding masking effects from the presence of fat.

The dissemination of gadopentetate dimeglumine into the extracellular space puts a premium on dynamic studies, and these have often been more revealing than static studies. The latter type of examination has failed to demonstrate major clinical advantages for contrast enhancement in a number of situations. Dynamic scanning may add significant new information.

In body applications, MRI is notable for the high tissue contrast available without enhancement. Gad-

opentetate dimeglumine is often of most value in specific clinical problems, such as improving the distinction between necrotic and viable tissue, helping differentiate benign from malignant tumors, and identifying recurrent tumor. Many of the initial studies have concentrated on tumor detection and differential diagnosis, reflecting the general field of application of MRI. A wider range of application is likely to be explored in the near future.

REFERENCES

1. Hamm B, Laniado M, Saini S. Contrast enhanced magnetic resonance imaging of the abdomen and pelvis. Magn Reson Q 1990;6:108–135.

2. Bloem JL, Reiser MF, Vanel D. Magnetic resonance contrast signals in the evaluation of the musculoskeletal system. Magn Reson Q 1990;6:136–163.

3. Saini S, Modic MT, Hamm B, Hahn PF. Advances in contrast enhanced MR imaging. AJR 1991;156:235–254.

4. Simon JH, Szumowski J. Chemical shift imaging with paramagnetic contrast enhancement for improved lesion depiction. Radiology 1989;171:539–543.

5. Mirowitz SA, Lee JKT, Gutierrez E, et al. Dynamic gadolinium enhanced rapid acquisition spin echo MR imaging of the liver. Radiology 1991;179:371–376.

6. Glazer GM, Gross BH, Aisen AM, et al. Imaging of the pulmonary hilum: a prospective study in patients with lung cancer. AJR 1985;145:245–248.

7. Grenier P, Dubray B, Corette MI, et al. Pre-operative thoracic staging of lung cancer. Diagn Intervent Radiol 1988;1:23–28.

8. Webb WR, Gatsonis C, Zouhouni EA, et al. CT and MR imaging in staging non-small cell bronchogenic carcinoma: report of the Radiologic Diagnostic Oncology Group. Radiology 1991;178:705–713.

9. Nishimura T, Kobayashi H, Okora Y, et al. General assessment of myocardial infarction by using gated MR imaging and gadopentetate dimeglumine. AJR 1989;153:715–720.

10. Eichstaedt HW, Felix R, Dougherty FC, et al. Magnetic resonance imaging (MRI) in different stages of myocardial infarction using the contrast agent gadolinium-DTPA. Clin Cardiol 1986;9:527–535.

11. Postenia S, de Roos A, Doornbos J, et al. Acute myocardial infarction: detection and localisation by magnetic resonance imaging and thallium. J Med Imaging 1989;3:68–74.

12. De Roos A, van Roosin AC, van der Wall EE, et al. Reperfused and non-reperfused myocardial infarction: value of gadolinium-DTPA enhanced MR imaging. Radiology 1989;172:717–720.

13. van der Wall EE, van Dykman PRM, de Roos A, et al. Diagnostic significance of gadolinium-DTPA enhanced magnetic resonance imaging on thrombolytic treatment for acute myocardial infarction: its potential in assessing reperfusion. Br Heart J 1990;63:12–17.

14. De Roos A, Matheijssen NAA, Doornbos J, et al. Myocardial infarct size after reperfusion therapy: assessment with gadopentetate dimeglumine enhanced MR imaging. Radiology 1990;176:517–521.

15. van Rugge FP, Boreel JJ, van Dijkman PRM, et al. Assessment of cardiac first-pass and myocardial perfusion using subsecond magnetic resonance imaging with gadolinium-DTPA. Abstracts 8th annual congress of the European Society for Magnetic Resononance in Medicine and Biology, Zurich, April 18–21. 1991:34.

16. Heywang SH, Hahn D, Schmidt H, et al. MR imaging of the breast using gadopentetate dimeglumine. J Comput Assist Tomogr 1986;10:199–204.

17. Heywang-Kobrunner SH. Contrast enhanced MRI of the breast. Munich: SH Karger, 1990.

18. Carr DH, Brown J, Bydder GM, et al. Gadolinium-DTPA as a contrast agent in MR: initial clinical experience in 20 patients. AJR 1984;143:215–224.

19. Hamm B, Wolf KJ, Felix R. Conventional and rapid MR imaging of the liver with gadolinium-DTPA. Radiology 1987;164:313–320.

20. Ohtumo K, Hai Y, Yoshikara K, et al. Hepatic tumors: dynamic MR imaging. Radiology 1987;163:27–31.

21. Hamm B, Fisher E, Taupite M. Differential of hepatic hemangioma from hepatic metastases by using dynamic contrast enhanced MR imaging. J Comput Assist Tomogr 1990;14:205–216.

22. Yosihida H, Hai Y, Ohtamara K, et al. Small hepatocellular carcinoma and hemangioma: differentiation with dynamic FLASH MR imaging with gadopentetate dimeglumine. Radiology 1989;171:339–342.

23. Pavone P, Giuliani S, Cardone G, et al. Intraarterial portography with gadopentetate dimeglumine: improved liver-to-lesion contrast in MR imaging. Radiology 1991;179:693–697.

24. Stark DD, Weissleder R, Elizendo G, et al. Superparamagnetic iron oxide: clinical application as a contrast agent for MR imaging of the liver. Radiology 1988;168:287–301.

25. Weissleder R, Stark DD, Rummeney EJ, et al. Splenic lymphoma: ferrite enhanced MR imaging in rats. Radiology 1988;166:423–430.

26. Hahn PF, Stark DD, Saini S, et al. Clinical trials of a superparamagnetic iron oxide gastrointestinal agent. Radiology 1990;175:695–700.

27. Lim KO, Stark DD, Leese PT, et al. Hepatobiliary MR imaging: first human experience with Mn DPDP. Radiology 1991;178:79–82.

28. Rummeny E, Stöber U, Wiesmann W, et al. Manganese-DPDP for enhanced detection and differential diagnosis of hepatic tumors. Abstracts 8th annual congress of the European Society for Magnetic Resonance in Medicine and Biology, Zurich, April 18–21. 1991:70.

29. Mirowitz SA, Brown JJ, Lee JKT, Heiken JP. Dynamic gadolinium-enhanced MR imaging of the spleen: normal enhancement patterns and evaluation of splenic lesions. Radiology 1991;179:681–686.

30. Maltry RF, Hajeck PC, Gylys-Monn V, et al. Perfluoro-chemicals and gastrointestinal agents for MR imaging: AJR 1987;148:1259–1263.

31. Laniado M, Kormmesser W, Hann B, et al. MR imaging of the gastrointestinal tract: value of Gd-DTPA. AJR 1988;150:817–821.

32. Hahn PF, Stark DD, Saini S, et al. Ferrite particles for bowel contrast in MR imaging: design issues and feasibility studies. Radiology 1987;164:37–40.

33. Lonnemark M, Hemmingsson A, Carlston J, et al. Superparamagnetic particles as an MRI contrast agent for the gastrointestinal tract. Acta Radiol 1988;29:599–602.

34. Lonnemark M, Hemmingsson A, Ericsson A, et al. The effect of oral superparamagnetic particles in plain and viscous aqueous suspensions. Acta Radiol 1990;29:303–307.

35. Choyke PL, Frank JA, Girton ME, et al. Dynamic gadolinium-DTPA enhanced MRI of the kidneys: a physiologic correlation. Radiology 1989;170:713–720.

36. Krestin P, Friedmann G, Steinbrich W, Linden A. Quantitative evaluation of renal function with rapid dynamic gadolinium-DTPA enhanced MRI. A comparison with radionuclide nephrography. Society of Magnetic Resonance in Medicine, 7th annual meeting, San Francisco, 1988.

37. Krestin GP, Friedmann G, Steinbrich W, Linden A. Gd-DTPA enhanced fast dynamic MRI of kidney and adrenals. Diagn Imaging 1988;4:40–44.

38. Patel SK, Stock CM, Turner DA. Magnetic resonance imaging in staging of renal cell carcinoma. Radiographics 1987;7:703–728.

39. Semelka RC, Hricak H, Stevens SK, et al. Combined gadolinium-enhanced and fat-saturation MR imaging of renal masses. Radiology 1991;178:803–809.

40. Reinig JW, Dopprain JL, Dwyer AJ, et al. Adrenal masses differentiated by MR. Radiology 1986;158:81–84.

41. Chang A, Glazer HS, Lee JKT, et al. Adrenal gland: MR imaging. Radiology 1987;163:123–128.

42. Falke THM, ter Strake L, Schaff MI, et al. MR imaging of the adrenals: correlation with computed tomography. J Comput Assist Tomogr 1986;10:242–253.

43. Krestin GP, Steinbrich W, Friedman G. Adrenal masses: evaluation with fast dynamic gradient echo MR imaging and gadopentetate dimeglumine enhanced dynamic studies. Radiology 1989;171:675–680.

44. Hricak H. MR of the female pelvis: review. AJR 1986;146:1115–1122.

45. Hricak H, Hamm B, Semelka R, et al. The use of gadopentetate dimeglumine in gynecologic oncology. Radiology 1991;(in press).

46. Mawhinney RR, Powell MC, Worthington BS, Symonds EM. Magnetic resonance imaging of benign ovarian masses. Br J Radiol 1988;61:179–186.

47. Chang YCF, Hricak H, Thurnher S, Carey CG. Evaluation of the vagina by magnetic resonance imaging. II. Neoplasm. Radiology 1988;160:431–435.

48. Johnson RJ, Carrington BM, Jenkins JPR, et al. Accuracy in staging carcinoma of the bladder by magnetic resonance imaging. Clin Radiol 1990;41;258–263.

49. Neuerburg JM, Bohndorf K, Sohn M, et al. Urinary bladder neoplasms: evaluation with contrast enhanced MR imaging. Radiology 1989;172:739–743.

50. Erlemann R, Reiser M, Peters PE, et al. Musculoskeletal neoplasms: static and dynamic gadopentetate dimeglumine MR imaging. Radiology 1989;171:767–773.

51. Erlemann R, Sciuk J, Bosse A, et al. Assessment of response to pre-operative chemotherapy in imaging osteosarcomas and Ewings sarcomas with dynamic and static skeletal scintigraphy. Radiology 1990;175:791–796.

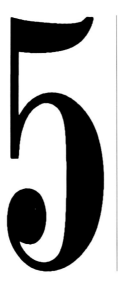

Future Directions in Magnetic Resonance Contrast Media

Val M. Runge

In less than a decade, magnetic resonance imaging (MRI) has come to occupy a major niche in diagnostic imaging, with the development of contrast agents helping to further expand clinical applications. Magnetic resonance imaging has the unique ability to obtain both high temporal and spatial resolution, with excellent sensitivity to contrast media. These characteristics, combined with high soft-tissue contrast and sensitivity to tissue abnormalities, have led to the replacement of x-ray computed tomography (CT) for patient diagnosis, particularly in the head, spine, and musculoskeletal system. Basic research is also being performed with magnetic resonance techniques, such as that available with positron emission tomography (PET) and single-photon emission computed tomography (SPECT), which provide biochemical and metabolic information concerning human disease. Newly developed techniques may provide a noninvasive, cost-effective means for elucidation of such basic physiologic information, with higher spatial resolution than is yet possible by other modalities. Rapid technological advances and extension of clinical applications, together with the innate chemical flexibility and potential offered by magnetic resonance imaging, are motivating the development of new MRI contrast agents.[1-4]

INTRAVENOUS AGENTS

Gadolinium Chelates

Clinical indications for intravenous injection of a gadolinium chelate are well established for head imaging.[5] Contrast enhancement is beneficial both for the visualization and characterization of space-occupying lesions. Enhancement occurs on the basis of either disruption of the blood–brain barrier or abnormal lesion vascularity. In particular, contrast enhancement permits visualization of small lesions, for example, meningiomas and intracanalicular acoustic neuromas, which can appear isointense relative to surrounding normal tissue on unenhanced scans.[6] Recurrent disease can also be quite difficult to differentiate from treatment-related changes without contrast administration.

Intravenous (IV) gadolinium chelate administration aids in the detection of extra-axial neoplasias, because of their vascularity, and in the detection of intra-axial neoplasia, owing to associated blood–brain barrier disruption. Visualization of arteriovenous malformations (AVMs) is improved because of vessel enhancement and increased flow-related artifacts. It is important to reemphasize that certain types of lesions, a prominent example being small metastatic foci, may be isointense on both precontrast T1- and T2-weighted images and also not elicit sufficient secondary changes to allow recognition, mandating the use of intravenous contrast agents, such as the gadolinium chelates, for lesion detection on MRI. For both intra-axial and extra-axial lesions, contrast enhancement often also proves valuable for the assessment of lesion extent. Gadolinium chelate administration has become standard for improved detection of pituitary microadenomas. Intravenous contrast enhancement has also been helpful in defining recurrent tumor in regions of previous surgery and in directing surgical biopsy.

With infection, IV gadolinium chelate administration improves both lesion detection and the assessment of disease activity (e.g., the differentiation of acute from chronic disease, or definition of disease progression in the face of antibiotic therapy). Sensitivity to all types of pathology in the posterior fossa or along the skull surpasses that of CT because of the absence of beam-

127

hardening artifacts with MRI. In normal patients, the falx and meninges do not become hyperintense following enhancement on MRI, unlike CT. Thus meningeal inflammatory or neoplastic disease is more easily detected on postcontrast MR scans. One pitfall for unenhanced MRI is the masking of certain peripheral or periventricular lesions by the high-signal intensity of adjacent cerebrospinal fluid (CSF) on T2-weighted examinations. Lesion recognition is possible, in this circumstance, by the enhancement of pathologic processes on postcontrast T1-weighted scans, owing to the large signal difference between enhancing lesions and low-signal intensity CSF.

Gadolinium chelate administration assists in the diagnosis of cerebral infarction. Subacute infarcts can be detected on the basis of blood–brain barrier disruption (typically visualized as gyriform enhancement), whereas luxury perfusion and venous stasis make possible dating and improve visualization of acute infarcts.

Indications for intravenous contrast administration in spinal examinations on MRI are, like the head, quite broad. Following surgery for disk herniation, contrast enhancement permits the differentiation of scar tissue (which enhances) from disk material (which does not enhance). This differential enhancement makes possible the diagnosis of recurrent or residual disk herniation in the back after surgery.[7,8] Contrast injection also aids in the visualization of drop metastases within the thecal sac and provides for the differentiation of neoplastic from congenital or traumatic syrinxes.[9] In certain instances, there may be improved visualization postcontrast of intrinsic cord lesions. The degree of enhancement found in spinal abnormalities is not always intense, suggesting the need for new contrast agents that would provide a greater change in T1 relaxation (either by greater intrinsic relaxivity enhancement or by improved safety, which would allow the use of higher doses).

More recently, clinical applications for the use of gadolinium chelates have been reported in musculoskeletal disease.[10] The extension of metastatic disease outside bone is well depicted on postcontrast scans, with good differentiation from surrounding normal soft tissue. Dynamic imaging performed immediately after contrast injection may improve the determination of a tumor's malignant potential by correlation with the initial rate of enhancement increase.[11] Lesion perfusion characteristics are also being used to predict response to chemotherapy. Gadolinium chelate injection has increased the specificity of MRI for cartilaginous tumors, affecting clinical management when tissue biopsy is technically difficult or inconclusive. Enhancement of inflamed synovium may be of value for the assessment of disease activity, as demonstrated in a report concerning MRI of the knee in rheumatoid arthritis.[12] Intra-articular (as opposed to intravenous) injection of a gadolinium chelate, although not approved for clinical use by the U.S. Food and Drug Administration (FDA), has improved the visualization and assessment of cartilaginous and tendon injuries, particularly for the rotator cuff and glenoid labrum.[13]

The use of intravenous gadolinium chelates is also being investigated in MRI of the chest, abdomen, and pelvis. Contrast enhancement can provide differentiation of infarcted from normal myocardium in cardiac imaging.[14] Administered in conjunction with fast-scanning techniques, liver perfusion can be studied within the first few minutes after injection.[15,16] Improved lesion detection could result from this approach. Differences in lesion perfusion characteristics could also potentially be exploited to improve lesion characterization: for example, in the differentiation of a malignant neoplasm from benign disease, such as focal nodular hyperplasia or hemangioma. The usefulness of intravenous gadolinium chelate administration in MRI of the spleen appears similar to that in the liver. Dynamic imaging during bolus contrast injection, in particular, may provide additional diagnostic information over unenhanced studies. The ability to enhance vascular structures is being exploited in MR angiography research.[17] Since these agents are excreted by glomerular filtration, improved differentiation of renal tumors from normal renal parenchyma may be possible, although initial results in this area have not been uniformly successful. Dynamic postcontrast renal imaging provides additional anatomic and functional information.

Growing clinical experience with gadopentetate dimeglumine and other gadolinium chelates has led to a discussion concerning the possible usefulness of higher doses of a contrast medium. The currently reported human studies with high-dose (greater than 0.1 mmol/kg) administration are summarized in Table 5–1. Gadopentetate dimeglumine has been evaluated at 0.2 mmol/kg in the brain,[18] liver,[19] breast,[20] and heart.[21] An increased "diagnostic yield" in selected intracranial tumors was noted with 0.2 mmol/kg. Improved enhancement of liver tumors has also been documented at this dose. However, gadopentetate dimeglumine has not been evaluated at doses higher than 0.1 mmol/kg in the United States or higher than 0.2 mmol/kg in Europe, possibly because of concerns relative to changes in blood chemistry following injection of higher doses. Other agents have been evaluated in patients at doses up to 0.4 mmol/kg.

In the head, it has been suggested that doses higher than 0.1 mmol/kg would be beneficial for identifying small (less than 1 to 2 mm) or poorly enhancing lesions. The use of lower doses (less than 0.1 mmol/kg) has not provided equivalent diagnostic information in controlled trials and has been motivated in part in the United States for financial reasons. In a study of intracranial tumors, the dose of 0.05 mmol/kg (gadopentetate dimeglumine) was diagnostically inadequate owing to the lack of distinct tumor-versus-brain contrast and inadequate tumor delineation.[22] In a study of intracranial metastatic disease, the dose of 0.3 mmol/kg (gadoteridol) improved lesion enhancement by 105%, compared with 0.1 mmol/kg, and permitted the identification of additional metastatic lesions on prospective scan interpretation.[23] The use of a high-contrast dose improved reader confidence in identification of metastatic lesions, permitted the identification of additional lesions, and excluded other lesions in question. Initial results also suggest that perfusion studies in the brain, made possible by newly available fast-imaging techniques, will be improved with administration of higher contrast doses.[24, 25]

In the spine, administration of high doses (more than 0.1 mmol/kg) should permit better visualization of vertebral body lesions and superior differentiation between scar and disk in the postsurgery patient. Studies in cardiac MRI suggest that it would be desirable to inject greater amounts of contrast medium to improve the distinction between acutely infarcted and normal, healthy myocardium. Abdominal imaging, particularly in the hepatic region, has been shown to be more diagnostic with higher contrast doses.[26] Studies have been pursued with both gadopentetate dimeglumine and gadoterate meglumine at a dose of 0.2 mmol/kg.[27] Early dynamic imaging following bolus contrast injection is likely to have a major impact on both lesion detection and characterization.[28–30] Experimental results in a liver abscess model confirm improved lesion depiction and detection at doses (gadoteridol) of 0.25 and 0.5 mmol/kg, compared with those of 0.1 mmol/kg.[31]

As requirements for increased dosage become apparent, work is being performed to develop new agents with improved tolerance so that high-dose applications will be possible. Increased emphasis is being placed on the physicochemical properties of the agents, such as osmolality and dissociation characteristics. Other investigators are attempting to solve the problem by improving the relaxivity of existing agents, thereby lowering the dose needed to produce increased enhancement. Both of these approaches seek to lower the toxicity of MRI contrast agents for a given effective dose. One step in development along these lines has paralleled the history of iodinated agents, with initial syntheses of ionic agents followed by production of nonionic or neutral agents.[32]

The clinical safety of gadolinium chelates is to a large extent dependent on the stability of the chelate in vivo. Key factors include thermodynamics, solubility, selectivity, and kinetics.[33,34] There must be a strong affinity between the metal ion and the chelate, reflected by the thermodynamic stability constant of the complex. The solubility of the complex can affect toxicity by possible precipitation of gadolinium ion. An important thermodynamic criterion is the selectivity of the chelate for the Gd^{3+} ion, as opposed to endogenous metal ions, in particular Zn^{2+}. And lastly, slow kinetics of dissociation can prevent release of gadolinium ion, lowering the toxicity, if clearance of the complex is sufficiently rapid.

The agents described subsequently fall into two basic groups, delineated by the type of chelate employed, which may be linear [based on diethylenetriamine pentaacetic acid (DTPA)] or macrocyclic. As previously noted, both the thermodynamic stability and the rate at which Gd^{3+} is released from the chelate in vivo are important determinants of safety. According to thermodynamic considerations and computer simulation of equilibria, administration of a slight excess of ligand for gadopentetate dimeglumine (and potentially other agents) should reduce interaction with metal ions that occur naturally in blood plasma.[35] For kinetic stability, macrocyclic polyazapolycarboxylate chelates demonstrate a distinct advantage.[36]

Gadopentetate Dimeglumine

Gadopentetate dimeglumine (Gd-DTPA; Magnevist, Berlex Laboratories, Cedar Knolls, New Jersey; Fig. 5–1A) was the first MRI contrast agent to be approved

(Text continues on page 132)

Table 5–1 **Worldwide High-Dose Experience (Humans)**

AGENT	APPLICATION	DATE	DOSE (mmol/kg)
Gadopentetate dimeglumine	Phase I	1983	≤ 0.25
	Brain (malignancy)	1987	0.2
	Liver (malignancy)	1989	0.2
	Breast	1989	0.2
	Heart (infarction)	1990	0.2
Gadoterate meglumine	Heart (infarction)	1991	0.4
Gadodiamide	Phase I	1988	≤ 0.3
Gadoteridol	Phase I	1989	≤ 0.3
	Phase II	1989	≤ 0.3
	Brain (metastases)	1990	0.3
	Liver	1991	0.3

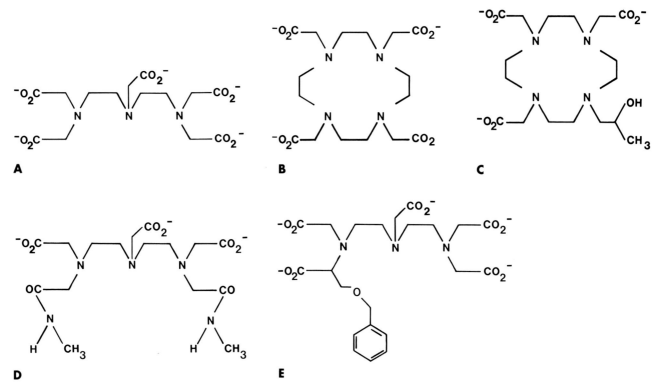

FIGURE 5-1 Chemical structure of the ligand for the gadolinium chelates in current clinical use or undergoing clinical evaluation. **(A)** diethylenetriaminepentaacetic acid (DPTA), the ligand in gadopentetate dimeglumine; **(B)** 1,4,7,10-tetraazacyclododecane tetraacetic acid (DOTA), the ligand in gadoterate meglumine; **(C)** 1,4,7-tris(carboxymethyl)-10-2'-hydroxypropyl)-1,4,7,10-tetraazacyclododecane (HP-DO3A), the ligand in gadoteridol; **(D)** diethylenetriaminepentaacetic acid bis-(methylamide) (DTPA-BMA), the ligand in gadodiamide; **(E)** BOPTA (DTPA with substitution of one proton from an acetate moiety by a benzyloxymethyl group).

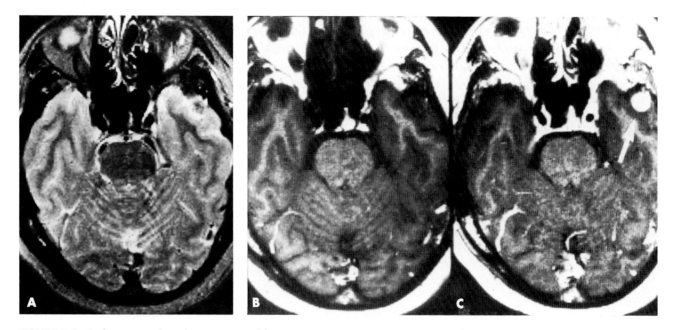

FIGURE 5-2 Gadopentetate dimeglumine: temporal fossa meningioma. **(A)** Precontrast T2-weighted and **(B, C)** pre- and postcontrast (0.1 mmol/kg IV) T1-weighted images employing gadopentetate dimeglumine. The lesion (arrow, **C**) is well depicted on the postcontrast examination owing to its vascularity. The lack of substantial mass effect or surrounding cerebral edema makes recognition difficult on precontrast images. (Reprinted with permission from Runge VM, ed. Clinical magnetic resonance imaging. Philadelphia: JB Lippincott, 1990)

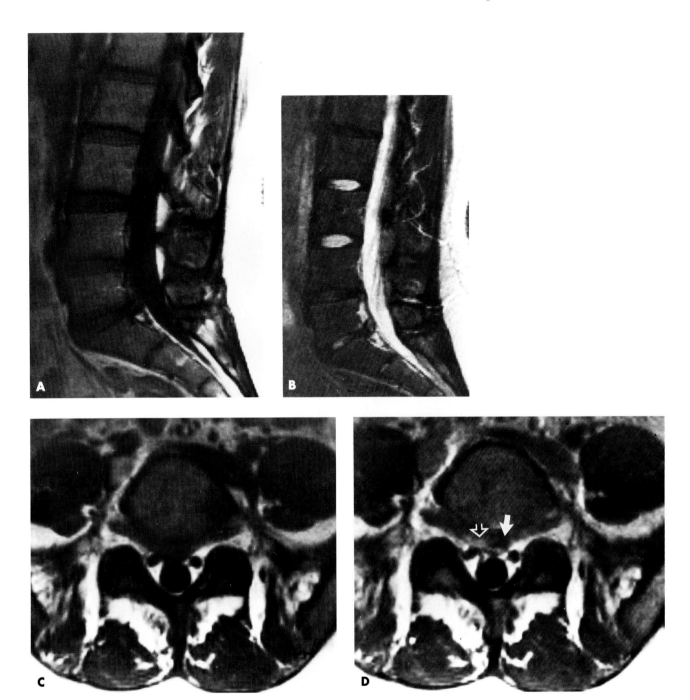

FIGURE 5-3 Gadopentetate dimeglumine: recurrent disk herniation in a 27-year-old woman who presented with increasing back pain and new right-sided radicular pain. **(A)** Sagittal T1-weighted and **(B)** T2-weighted images; **(C, D)** pre- and immediate postgadopentetate dimeglumine (0.1 mmol/kg IV) axial T1-weighted images. A recurrent central disk herniation (which does not enhance; *white arrow,* **D**) can be differentiated from postoperative fibrosis (which does enhance; *open arrow,* **D**) by the vascular nature of scar. (Reprinted with permission from Runge VM, ed. Clinical magnetic resonance imaging. Philadelphia: JB Lippincott, 1990)

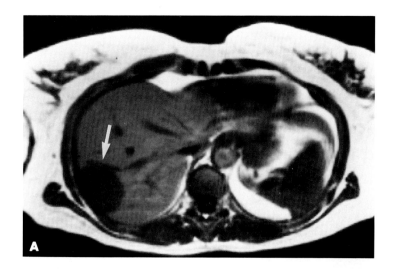

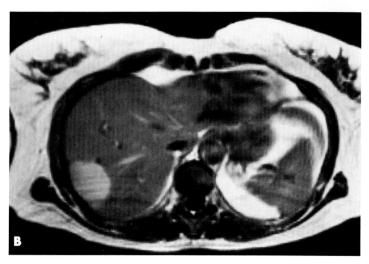

FIGURE 5-4 Gadopentetate dimeglumine: cavernous hemangioma. T1-weighted axial spin echo nonbreathhold images acquired **(A)** before and **(B)** after gadopentetate dimeglumine injection (0.1 mmol/kg IV). This highly vascular lesion (*arrow*, **A**) enhances to a greater extent than the surrounding normal hepatic tissue, improving diagnostic specificity. (Reprinted with permission from Runge VM, ed. Clinical magnetic resonance imaging. Philadelphia: JB Lippincott, 1990)

by the FDA for clinical use (June 1988).[37] Gadopentetate dimeglumine is approved for use in the general population aged 2 years and older for examinations of the head (Fig. 5–2) and spine (Fig. 5–3), at a dose of 0.1 mmol/kg.[38–40] Clinical trials are also now complete in the neck, oropharynx, and nasopharynx[41] in the United States. Extensive clinical experience has been gained with this agent outside of the central nervous system (CNS) in recent years, particularly for body (Fig. 5–4) and musculoskeletal imaging. Relative contraindications exist for gadopentetate dimeglumine use in patients with hemolytic anemias or impaired renal function. The former restriction arose because of the elevation in serum iron concentrations observed during clinical trials; the latter restriction because of the primary excretion of the agent by glomerular filtration. Limited studies in patients with chronic renal failure have demonstrated no change in serum creatinine levels in long-term follow-up after contrast administration. It has also been shown that gadopentetate dimeglumine can be eliminated by hemodialysis; three dialysis treat-

ments given within 5 days resulted in 97% clearance of the agent.[42] Laboratory abnormalities are known following gadopentetate dimeglumine administration. In a study by Goldstein and co-workers, 11% of men (34 of 308) had abnormal serum iron levels and 2.9% (11 of 379) abnormal bilirubin levels at 24 hours postcontrast. In healthy volunteers, after a dose of 0.25 mmol/kg, the changes in serum iron and total bilirubin levels could be observed at 3 to 4 hours, were maximum at 6 to 12 hours, and returned to baseline values by 24 hours.[43] These results appear to be of no clinical consequence and can be explained by slight hemolysis after the IV contrast injection. The effect of the agent (or for that matter any gadolinium chelate) on the developing fetus or newborn is unknown; therefore, gadopentetate dimeglumine is not recommended for use in pregnant or lactating women.[44] Following the first year of its clinical use, there was a 3% rate of reported adverse reactions, the majority considered mild by reporting physicians (hives, nausea, headaches, pain, or a cold sensation at the injection site) and only

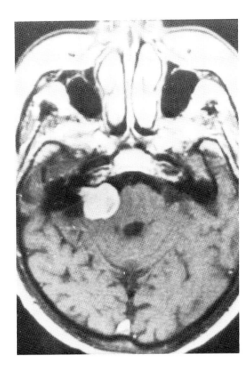

FIGURE 5-5 Gadoterate meglumine: right cerebello-pontine angle acoustic neuroma. Axial postgadoterate meglumine (0.1 mmol/kg IV) T1-weighted image. Enhancement of this extra-axial lesion permits improved boundary demarcation and anatomic localization, with extension of the tumor into the internal auditory canal well delineated postcontrast. (Reprinted with permission from Runge VM, ed. Enhanced magnetic resonance imaging. St Louis: CV Mosby, 1989)

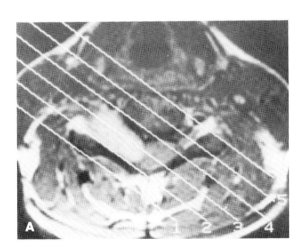 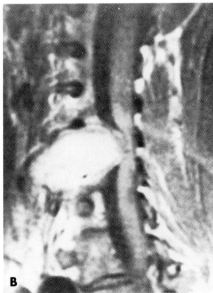

FIGURE 5-6 Gadoterate meglumine: right C5-6 cervical neuroma. Axial **(A)** and oblique sagittal **(B)** T1-weighted images through the right C5-6 vertebral foramen following injection of gadoterate meglumine (0.1 mmol/kg IV). Contrast enhancement allows differentiation of tumor, bone, and soft tissue. The oblique planes acquired are indicated on the axial image. (Reprinted with permission from Runge VM, ed. Enhanced magnetic resonance imaging. St Louis: CV Mosby, 1989)

two described as moderate (seizures, vomiting).[45] Caution should be exercised with bolus injection, particularly considering the restrictive nature of the magnet bore in most MRI installations, given the reports of emesis (12 of 4260 patients).[46] Administration of gadopentetate dimeglumine, as with all intravenous contrast media, should be overseen by a physician, particularly in view of recently described severe anaphylactic-type reactions.[47]

Gadoterate Meglumine

In early 1989, a second contrast agent, gadoterate meglumine (Gd-DOTA; Dotarem, Laboratoire Guerbet, Aulnay-sous-Bois, France; see Fig. 5–1B) was approved for initial clinical use. To date, gadoterate meglumine has been used in more than 53,000 patients and is approved in France, Portugal, Belgium, Switzerland, and Brazil (approval is pending in Holland). The recommended dose (IV) is 0.1 mmol/kg. The chelate (DOTA) in this instance has a macrocyclic structure, as opposed to the linear structure of DTPA. Rigid macrocyclic complexes such as Gd-DOTA demonstrate improved stability in vivo owing to slow dissociation kinetics.[48] Gadoterate meglumine, like gadopentetate dimeglumine, is an extracellular agent that is administered intravenously. Because of similarities in relaxivity and distribution, applications for gadoterate meglumine[49] (Figs. 5–5 and 5–6) should prove similar to those for gadopentetate dimeglumine. Investigation is under way with gadoterate meglumine in applications using doses higher than 0.1 mmol/kg.[50] The injection of gadoterate meglumine has no known effect upon serum iron levels. In a study of 4169 patients receiving gadoterate meglumine,[51] no life-threatening event was reported, and one or more adverse reactions were reported in 0.8%. Vomiting was noted in 8 patients postcontrast. Plasma pharmacokinetics appear similar to gadopentetate dimeglumine. In a study of normal volunteers, the plasma elimination half-life was 91 ± 14 minutes and the distribution volume was 171 ± 20

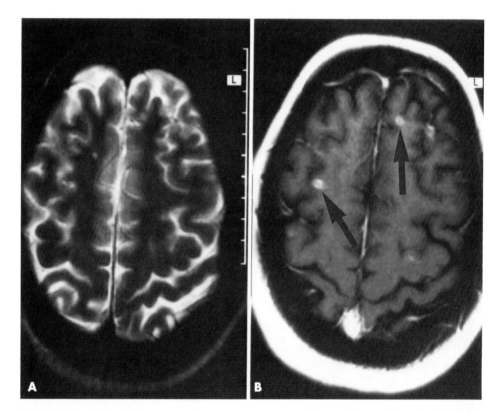

FIGURE 5-7 Gadoteridol: metastatic breast carcinoma in a 31-year-old woman. Axial **(A)** precontrast T2-weighted and **(B)** postcontrast T1-weighted images employing gadoteridol at a dose of 0.1 mmol/kg IV. In this patient, a diagnosis of intracerebral metastatic disease was possible only following contrast enhancement. Seven lesions were identified on the postcontrast images [two are depicted with *arrows* **(B)** on the section presented], each appearing isointense on the corresponding precontrast T1- and T2-weighted examinations. The isointensity of the lesions, together with the lack of mass effect or accompanying cerebral edema, resulted in the precontrast scans being interpreted as within normal limits (specifically no evidence of metastatic disease). (Reprinted with permission from Runge VM, et al. Clinical safety and efficacy of gadoteridol (Gd HP-DO3A)—a study of 411 patients with suspected intracranial and spinal pathology. Radiology 1991; in press)

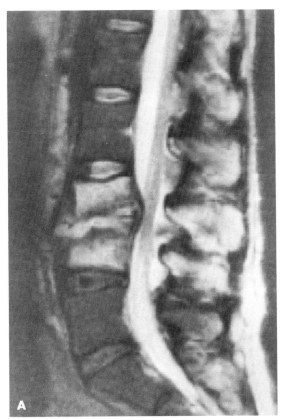

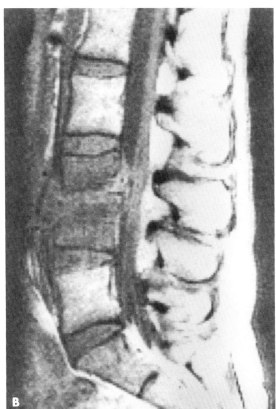

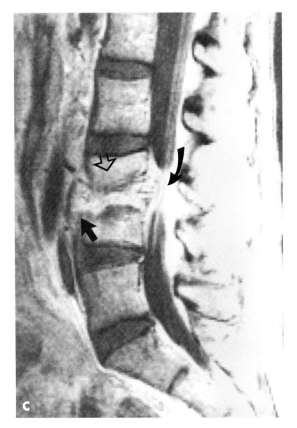

FIGURE 5-8 Gadoteridol: staphylococcal osteomyelitis involving L3-4 in a 42-year-old patient. Sagittal **(A)** T2-weighted, **(B)** precontrast T1-weighted, and **(C)** postgadoteridol injection (0.1 mmol/kg IV) T1-weighted images. Contrast enhancement is present both within the vertebral body (*open arrow,* **C**), consistent with osteomyelitis, and within the paraspinous soft tissue mass (*solid arrow,* **C**). Enhancement also improves the depiction of thecal sac compression (*curved arrow,* **C**) by the extradural mass.

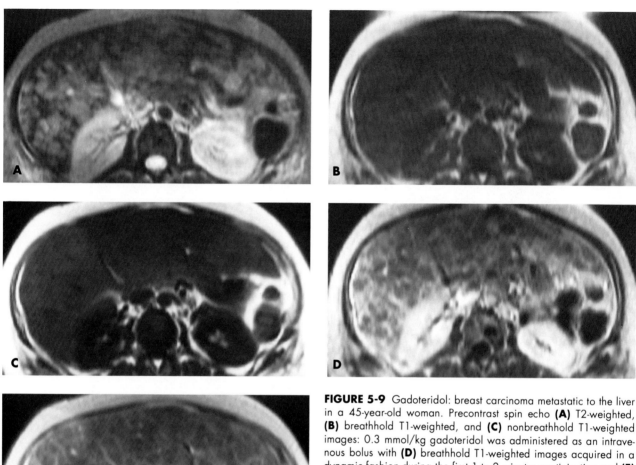

FIGURE 5-9 Gadoteridol: breast carcinoma metastatic to the liver in a 45-year-old woman. Precontrast spin echo **(A)** T2-weighted, **(B)** breathhold T1-weighted, and **(C)** nonbreathhold T1-weighted images: 0.3 mmol/kg gadoteridol was administered as an intravenous bolus with **(D)** breathhold T1-weighted images acquired in a dynamic fashion during the first 1 to 2 minutes postinjection and **(E)** nonbreathhold T1-weighted images acquired at approximately 5 minutes postinjection. Diffuse metastatic disease in the liver in this case causes the heterogenous appearance on T2-weighted images, with unenhanced T1-weighted images being nondiagnostic. Following high-dose contrast administration, both dynamic and static T1-weighted images reveal differential enhancement for metastatic tumor (of lower signal intensity) and the small amount of residual normal liver (of higher signal intensity postcontrast, enhancing to a greater degree than neoplastic tissue).

mL/kg. These results are consistent with rapid passive distribution in the interstitial space, followed by rapid urinary excretion by glomerular filtration.[52]

Gadoteridol

Gadoteridol (Gd-HP-DO3A[53]; ProHance, Squibb Diagnostics, Princeton, New Jersey; see Fig. 5–1C) has been studied in more than 500 patients, with approval for clinical use at a dose of 0.1 mmol/kg IV pending in the United States. Clinical trials are also in progress in Europe and Japan. Gadoteridol is a macrocyclic, neutral (zero net charge), extracellular chelate,[54] with safety demonstrated at doses up to 0.3 mmol/kg[55] in Phase II and III United States clinical trials. Like gadoterate meglumine, gadoteridol is relatively inert to metal ion substitution (Zn^{2+}, Cu^{2+}, and Ca^{2+} transmetallation),[56,57] when compared with gadopentetate dimeglumine. Since

in vivo dissociation, yielding free metal ion and ligand, is one mechanism of toxicity for gadolinium chelates, the greater kinetic stability of such rigid macrocyclic structures may lead to improved safety. As with gadopentetate dimeglumine, space-occupying lesions within the central nervous system that have caused blood–brain barrier disruption (Fig. 5–7) or that are characterized by a large vascular supply demonstrate significant enhancement following gadoteridol injection. Applications for gadoteridol in the spine, similar to those of gadopentetate dimeglumine, include the differentiation of residual or recurrent disk herniation from postoperative change, improved characterization of and sensitivity to infectious processes (Fig. 5–8), identification of drop metastases, and determination of the soft tissue neoplastic extent. Animal research has demonstrated efficacy of gadoteridol at higher doses

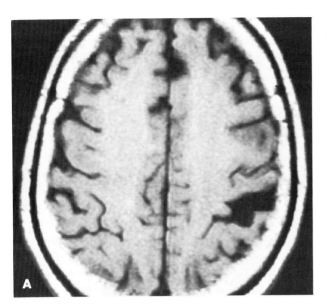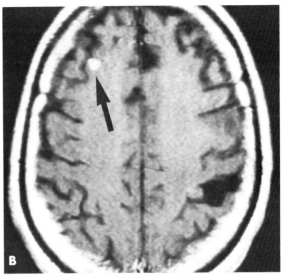

FIGURE 5-10 Gadodiamide: metastatic lung carcinoma. T1-weighted axial images **(A)** before and **(B)** after IV injection of gadodiamide (0.1 mmol/kg). A single metastatic lesion (*arrow,* **B**) can be seen following contrast administration. This was not noted prospectively on unenhanced T1- or T2- (not shown) weighted scans. (Courtesy of Salutar Inc, Sunnyvale, California)

(0.3 to 0.5 mmol/kg) for dynamic liver imaging, cardiac imaging, and brain perfusion studies (personal communication, Squibb Diagnostics, New Brunswick, New Jersey). Gadoteridol is unique among the gadolinium chelates in that doses up to 0.3 mmol/kg have been investigated in both brain and liver imaging (clinical trials in both areas are currently in progress). Clinical results, although preliminary, indicate definite clinical efficacy for high-contrast dose in certain patient populations in both brain (see Chap. 2) and liver (Fig. 5–9) neoplastic disease.

In a Phase III trial of 411 patients,[58] adverse events possibly or probably related to administration of contrast material occurred in 4% of all patients, with the majority mild in intensity. The overall incidence of adverse reactions with gadoteridol appears similar to that with gadopentetate dimeglumine. No clinically remarkable laboratory abnormalities have been observed following gadoteridol administration, unlike gadopentetate dimeglumine, which is associated with changes in serum iron and bilirubin levels. No emesis has been observed with bolus administration in limited clinical experience.

Gadodiamide

Gadodiamide (Gd-DTPA-BMA; Omniscan, Salutar Inc., Sunnyvale, California and Winthrop Pharmaceuticals, New York, New York; see Fig. 5–1D) is a neutral gadolinium chelate that has been evaluated in clinical trials in the United States and Europe and was recently submitted to the FDA for clinical approval. The ligand

itself (DTPA-BMA) is a derivative of DTPA, with neutrality achieved by replacement of two of the anionic donors (CO^{2-}) with methylamides. Removal of the acid groups leads to a significant decrease in the thermodynamic stability constant for the complex (log K_{Therm} = 16.85 for gadodiamide as opposed to 22.46 for Na_2 [Gd-DTPA]). The pharmaceutical composition of gadodiamide contains 5% calcium DTPA-BMA (mole/mole). Questions have been raised concerning delayed death in acute toxicology studies (in animals) and overall product tolerance [Discussion section, Workshop on Contrast Enhanced Magnetic Resonance Imaging (Society of Magnetic Resonance in Medicine) 1991, Napa, California and personal communication, D. Meyer, Laboratoire Guerbet]. Patient trials have shown the usefulness of enhancement with gadodiamide on MRI examinations of the CNS.[59,60] No substantial differences in enhancement characteristics (Figs. 5–10 and 5–11) have been described relative to gadopentetate dimeglumine. Gadodiamide was studied at dosages up to 0.3 mmol/kg in Phase I, with no clinically significant adverse events reported. In a study of 73 patients at 0.1 mmol/kg,[59] there were marked abnormalities in serum iron levels in 6 (8%), yet no similar changes in bilirubin levels. In Phase II/III investigation at 15 centers, 439 patients were evaluated following a dose of 0.1 mmol/kg IV (personal communication, Salutar Inc., Sunnyvale, California). The most common adverse events were mild to moderate headache (3.4%), dizziness (1.8%), and nausea (1.6%). Approximately half of the headaches were not considered related to drug administration.

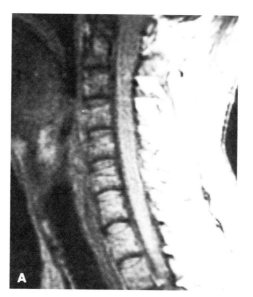 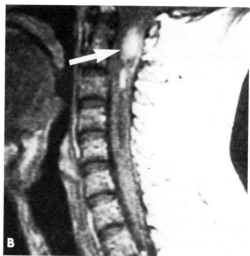

FIGURE 5-11 Gadodiamide: cord astrocytoma. Sagittal T1-weighted scans **(A)** pre- and **(B)** post-gadodiamide injection (0.1 mmol/kg IV). Enhancement can be noted in portions of this cervicomedullary junction astrocytoma (*arrow*, **B**), distinguishing this lesion from a benign syrinx. (Courtesy Salutar Inc, Sunnyvale, California)

Gadopenamide

Gadopenamide (Gd-DTPA bismorpholide; Schering AG, Berlin)[61] is a low osmolar linear gadolinium chelate with excellent tolerance demonstrated in animal studies. In higher dose applications (>0.1 mmol/kg), benefits from this type of agent could be significant.

Gadolinium MCTA

Gadolinium methyl 2-1,4,7,10-tetraazacyclododecane-N,N',N'', N'''-tetraacetic acid (Gd-MCTA; Laboratoire Guerbet, Aulnay-sous-Bois, France), like Gd-DOTA, is characterized by a very slow rate of formation (high kinetic stability). MCTA is similar to DOTA in chemical structure, with the addition of a methylene group on the ethylene bridge. However, Gd-MCTA exhibits a significantly lower toxicity,[62] as assessed by the 50% lethal dose (LD_{50}) measurements in mice. The LD_{50} reported for Gd-MCTA was 15 mmol/kg versus 11.2 mmol/kg for Gd-DOTA.[63] This improved tolerance may be the result of slower dissociation kinetics, with additional rigidity provided by steric hindrance of the methyl group. The relaxivity characteristics of Gd-MCTA and Gd-DOTA are quite similar. Further investigation of this compound is in progress.

Gadolinium BOPTA Dimeglumine

Gadolinium BOPTA (Gd-DTPA-benzyloxymethyl; Bracco Industria Chimica SpA, Milan, Italy; see Fig. 5–1E)[64,65] is an extracellular agent with both biliary and urinary excretion. Animal studies have demonstrated prolonged hepatic enhancement, with high and persistent liver–tumor contrast on MRI. In myocardial imaging, greater and more persistent signal intensity enhancement (using contrast-to-noise ratio measurements) of normal myocardium relative to acute infarction has been demonstrated compared with that of gadopentetate dimeglumine. Enhancement of normal liver in humans has been demonstrated in Phase I trials.

Gadolinium Ethoxybenzyl Diethylenetriamine Pentaacetate Disodium

Gadolinium ethoxybenzyl-DTPA[66] (Gd-EOB-DTPA; Schering AG, Berlin, Germany)- is a lipophilic agent, with high water solubility and low toxicity (LD_{50} = 7.5 mmol/kg). The distribution of the agent is extracellular, other than in the liver. Because of its protein binding (10%), negative charge, and lipophilic nature, Gd-EOB-DTPA exhibits both renal (30%) and hepatobiliary (70%) excretion. Uptake into hepatocytes is through an anionic carrier-mediated transport mechanism. T1 relaxivity was measured to be 5.3 L $mmol^{-1} \cdot s^{-1}$ in water. Similar to other liver-specific paramagnetic compounds, T1 relaxivity in liver is markedly increased (16.9 L $mmol^{-1} \cdot s^{-1}$), presumably by protein binding, higher viscosity, or reduced mobility of the compound. Optimal enhancement occurs shortly after injection. Specific applications for both cholangiography and enhanced detection of hepatic metastases have been demonstrated in animal models. Compounds such as Gd-EOB-DTPA or Gd-BOPTA could also function as conventional extracellular contrast agents, in addition to providing liver enhancement.

Nongadolinium Chelates

An alternative route being investigated is the development of contrast agents that are specially targeted to organ systems or by tissue function. Within this class lie agents directed at hepatocytes, the reticuloendothelial system (RES), and the circulating blood pool. Gadopentetate dimeglumine and the majority of new intravenous agents now completing clinical trials distribute to the extracellular space and depend primarily upon glomerular filtration for excretion. The idea behind specifically targeting agents is to limit the areas to which the contrast medium will go and thus cause more tissue-specific or disease-directed enhancement. This is particularly important in areas, such as the abdomen, where lesions of the liver and spleen may actually appear less distinct following administration of an extracellular agent—especially when standard doses (0.1 mmol/kg of gadopentetate dimeglumine) and imaging techniques (nondynamic) are employed. Two gadolinium-based chelates just discussed, Gd-BOPTA dimeglumine and Gd-EOB-DTPA disodium, were actually designed according to this approach, with preferential hepatobiliary excretion and, thus, hepatic enhancement.

Agents that selectively accumulate within a certain tissue or organ of interest can substantially improve detection of abnormality or disease.[67,68] Targeting can be achieved by altering particle size, or by binding paramagnetic (or superparamagnetic) agents to molecules that have a selective distribution, either because of size or receptor binding. Additional approaches include the covalent linkage of paramagnetic agents to macromolecules (e.g., dextran),[69] or encapsulation (entrapping) in liposomes, thereby changing their distribution. When covalently linked, an additional result is an increase in relaxivity owing to the increase in the correlation time of rotation. But this is also typically accompanied by a decrease in the conditional stability constant and, thus, an increase in the risk for dissociation.

A different avenue for contrast agent development is represented by dysprosium (Dy) chelates, which may find application for the assessment of tissue perfusion by measurement of changes in magnetic susceptibility immediately following bolus contrast injection. Such compounds would act as "negative" contrast agents, creating by their presence in vivo a small localized magnetic field gradient, thereby causing a decrease in the signal intensity observed on MRI in perfused tissue. Experimental animal investigations with Dy-DTPA-BMA have confirmed the ability of MRI to evaluate both myocardial[70] and brain[71] perfusion by this dynamic susceptibility contrast approach.

Manganese Dipyridoxyl Diphosphate

Manganese dipyridoxyl diphosphate (Mn-DPDP; Salutar Inc., Sunnyvale, California; Fig. 5–12) was developed specifically for hepatobiliary MRI. The DPDP ligand was designed to be recognized by the membrane transport system in the liver for the coenzyme pyridoxal-5′-phosphate, one of the B_6 vitamin complex. The agent is distributed both extracellularly and intracellularly, and is actively taken up by hepatocytes in normal liver. Manganese DPDP enhances normal hepatic tissue, enabling potentially improved focal lesion detection (as lower signal intensity abnormalities) and assessment of liver function (Fig. 5–13). Clearance is by both renal and hepatic pathways. In preclinical evaluation, T1 relaxivity was 2.8 $[mmol/L]^{-1}\cdot s^{-1}$, of similar magnitude to gadopentetate dimeglumine = 4.5 $[mmol/L]^{-1}\cdot s^{-1}$, and increased in liver tissue to 21.7 $[mmol/L]^{-1}\cdot s^{-1}$. Maximum liver enhancement was observed at 30 minutes postinjection, with 13% of the agent in liver at that time.[72] The LD_{50}/effective dose (at 10 μmol/kg), one measure of safety, was determined to be 540, substan-

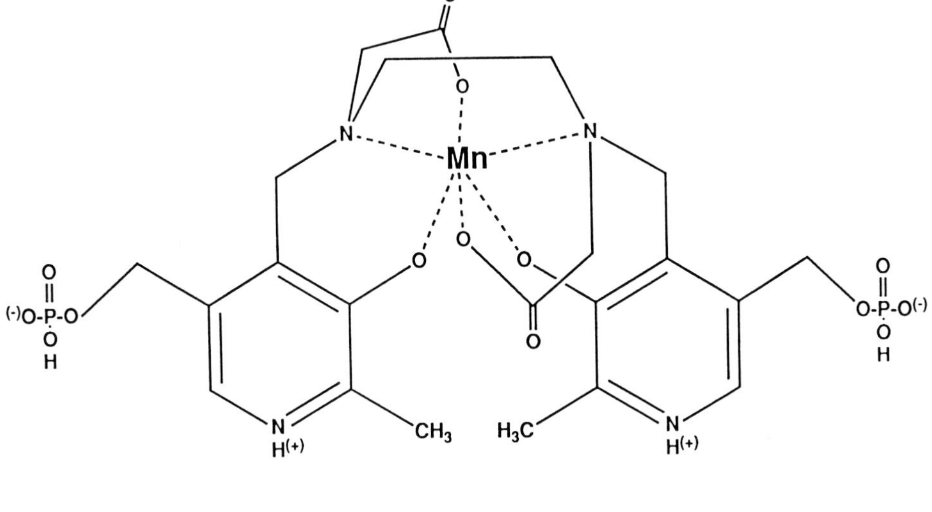

FIGURE 5-12 Mn-DPDP (manganese [II] N,N′-dipyridoxylethylenediamine-N,N′-diacetate-5,5′-bis[phosphate]). (Courtesy of Salutar Inc, Sunnyvale, California)

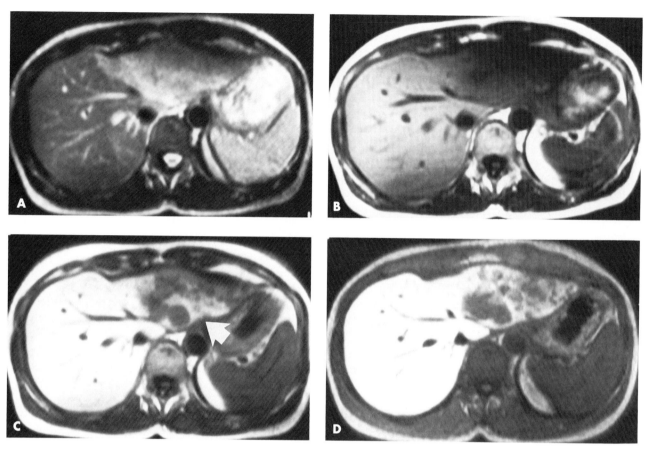

FIGURE 5-13 Mn DPDP: hepatocellular carcinoma in the left lobe of the liver. Precontrast **(A)** T2-(TR/TE = 2000/70) and **(B)** T1- (TR/TE = 500/15) weighted spin echo images; postcontrast T1-weighted **(C)** spin echo and **(D)** gradient echo (TR/TE/tip angle = 100/6/60°) images 30 minutes after IV injection of 10 μmol/kg Mn DPDP. The area of abnormality is slightly larger on precontrast T2-weighted, as opposed to T1-weighted images, consistent with a component of edema. Contrast enhancement reveals multiple nonenhancing nodular abnormalities in the left hepatic lobe (*arrow*, **C**), improving lesion visualization and the differentiation of neoplastic tissue from normal liver and edema. Note the substantial enhancement of normal liver postcontrast. (Courtesy of Dr. E. Rummeny, University of Muenster, Germany)

tially higher than that for gadopentetate dimeglumine (60 to 100). Phase I and II clinical trials have been completed in the United States. In initial human investigation, 12 normal volunteers received doses of 3, 10, or 15 μmol/kg. Normal liver demonstrated a 75% to 100% signal enhancement 10 minutes after injection of 10 μmol/kg.[73]

Although the number of subjects studied was small (four at 10 μmol/kg and three at 15 μmol/kg), there appeared to be no difference in liver parenchyma enhancement between the 10- and 15-μmol/kg doses, with saturation of cellular uptake mechanisms a possible explanation (personal communication, Salutar Inc., Sunnyvale, California). Facial flushing has been observed with contrast administration (≤10 μmol/kg) and transient hypertension at doses higher than 10 μmol/kg.[74] In Phase II in the United States, four different doses

(3, 5, 8, and 10 μmol/kg) were given to 96 patients, with half receiving the contrast as a bolus and half as an infusion. Preliminary results demonstrate improved delineation of tumors from normal liver tissue postcontrast and an increased rate of detection of small tumors (<1.5 cm). Enhancement of the pancreas and kidneys was also noted. One possible advantage for Mn-DPDP, when compared with gadolinium chelates without preferential hepatobiliary excretion, is the prolonged window (at least several hours, compared with just minutes during bolus administration of a gadolinium chelate) for diagnostic imaging. Animal experimentation has demonstrated efficacy for improved detection of liver metastases (using a dose of 50 μmol/kg)[75]; assessment of hepatocyte function and detection of early hepatocyte necrosis (using a dose of 50 μmol/kg)[76]; delineation of acute myocardial ischemia (using a dose of 400 μmol/kg)[77]; and potentially the discrimination between reperfused and occlusive myocardial infarction.[78]

Iron (III) Ethylenebis-(2-hydroxyphenyl)glycine

Iron (III) ethylenebis-(2-hydrophenyl)glycine (Fe-EHPG) has been investigated for possible use to improve visualization of small metastatic lesions within the liver.[79] In two models of liver tumors in mice, at a dose of 0.1 mmol/kg, Fe-EHPG improved visualization of smaller (≤5 mm) metastatic lesions. Postcontrast images were superior for lesion detection to precontrast T1- and T2-weighted images, using liver-to-tumor contrast-to-noise (C/N) ratios for quantitation. Liver-to-tumor C/N improved by more than a factor of 4 when comparing preinjection and postinjection T1-weighted images. Derivatives of Fe-EHPG, as well as other iron chelates (e.g., Fe-HBED), have also been investigated.[80]

Particulate Agents

Particulate agents containing iron oxide, as designed for use in MRI, fall within four classes: conventional superparamagnetic iron oxide, ultrasmall iron oxide preparations, receptor-directed iron oxide, and antibody-labeled iron oxide.[81] Conventional agents include magnetite (alone or coated with albumin or dextran), ferromagnetic microspheres (in a starch or albumin matrix), and dextran-coated polycrystalline iron oxides. These compounds have a short in vivo half-life (< 15 minutes) and demonstrate predominate uptake in the liver and spleen from phagocytosis by the reticuloendothelial system (RES). Of these agents, AMI-25 has been most extensively evaluated. A similar compound, magnetic starch microspheres (MSM, iron oxide crystals embedded in hydrolyzed starch) is under development by Nycomed (personal communication, Nycomed AS Imaging, Oslo, Norway). Ultrasmall (<20 nm) iron oxides demonstrate a longer in vivo half-life (>40 minutes) and can leave the vascular system (because of their size) by vesicular transport or through endothelial junctions. Thus, these particles are also taken up by macrophages in lymph nodes and bone marrow. Major applications include imaging of the lymphatic system and bone marrow. Ultrasmall iron oxide particles can also be coupled to receptor-specific carrier molecules, an approach that has been investigated with the asialoglycoprotein (ASG) receptor system. The ASG receptor system on hepatocytes was chosen for initial investigation, since it is well characterized, with a large number of ligand-binding sites per cell, and can be easily targeted by attaching terminal galactose sugars to the desired pharmaceutical agent. To successfully develop antibody-labeled iron oxide, very small (<10 nm) superparamagnetic tracer compounds had to be developed that would not be rapidly taken up by macrophages and that could pass through capillary fenestrae or endothelial junctions, or be transported by vesicles, to reach the extravascular space. Monocrystalline iron oxide nanopolymer (MION) fulfills these criteria and has been successfully coupled to antimyosin. A monoclonal antibody to colon carcinoma has also been successfully attached to magnetite (Fe_3O_4) particles (average core size ≈ 10 nm), with retention of immunoreactivity and MR relaxation properties.[82]

AMI-25

Particulate imaging agents that are cleared by the reticuloendothelial elements of the liver, spleen, and bone marrow have long been used in nuclear medicine to detect space-occupying liver lesions that displace Kupffer cells. AMI-25 (Advanced Magnetics Inc, Cambridge, Massachusetts) is composed of biodegradable, superparamagnetic iron oxide particulates with a mean diameter of 80 nm, as measured by laser light scattering.[83] After IV injection, the agent is rapidly cleared from the circulation by reticuloendothelial system (RES) phagocytosis; the iron is metabolically degraded over a few days and enters the marrow for red blood cell synthesis. In animal investigation, peak iron concentration was observed in the liver after 2 hours and in the spleen after 4 hours, with no acute or subacute toxic effects detected by histologic or serologic studies.[84] The presence of iron oxide in tissue produces a large decrease in T2, causing normal liver to have significantly reduced signal intensity on MRI.[85,86] This characteristic contrast-agent-induced reduction in tissue signal intensity has led to categorization of AMI-25 and related agents as negative contrast media. Since most liver lesions, including tumors, cysts, and abscesses, have no RES components, they do not take up the imaging agent and appear bright against the darkened background of normal tissue (Fig. 5–14). Unfortunately, impaired uptake of AMI-25 has been demonstrated in rats treated with CCl_4 (which causes impairment of Kupffer cell phagocytic function), casting doubt upon the diagnostic efficacy of this agent in patients with severe cirrhosis.[87]

Clinical experience has demonstrated significantly increased tumor-to-liver contrast-to-noise ratios after AMI-25 administration, which permitted detection of hepatic lesions as small as 3 to 5 mm in diameter. In the pilot study of 15 patients, doses of 10 to 50 μmol/kg were administered.[88] Two drug-related adverse reactions were observed, transient hypotension and rash, each in one patient. Small blood vessels with slow flow, imaged in cross section, can be difficult to distinguish from small metastatic lesions following AMI-25 administration, with both appearing hyperintense. Dynamic imaging may be helpful in this distinction by elucidating differences in perfusion or bulk blood flow. In a second

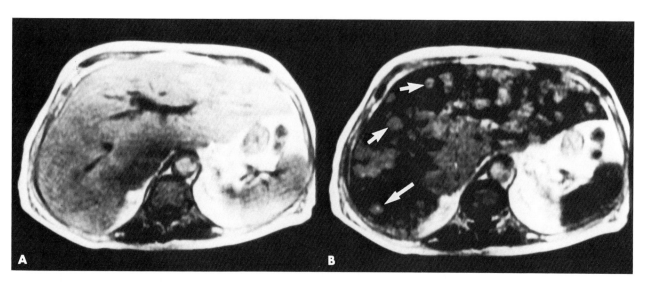

FIGURE 5-14 AMI-25: multiple hepatic metastases. T2-weighted (TR/TE = 1500/40) images **(A)** before and **(B)** after injection of AMI-25 (Fe, 20 μmol/kg). Following contrast administration, the signal intensity of normal liver tissue is markedly reduced, improving visualization of multiple intrahepatic lesions (*arrows*, **B**). (Courtesy of Advanced Magnetics Inc, Cambridge, Massachusetts)

study of 19 patients,[89] imaging was performed both during the distribution phase (within 12 minutes of injection) and the retention phase (1 to 2 hours after injection) of the contrast agent. Ninety percent of lesions could be demonstrated on the distribution phase images, with increased diagnostic confidence from the reduction of signal intensity of small blood vessels imaged in cross section. As with all RES agents, the differential diagnosis of space-occupying lesions demonstrated by AMI-25 must take into account the possibility of focal nodular hyperplasia, benign adenomas, abscesses, cysts, and hemangiomas, as well as metastatic deposits. Because of its splenic uptake, AMI-25 has been used as an adjunct to the diagnosis of splenic metastases[90] and diffuse infiltration by lymphoma.[91] As a consequence of markedly improved tumor–spleen contrast-to-noise ratio following AMI-25 administration, splenic tumors were identified in 4 of 18 patients, compared with 2 of 18 patients precontrast. In splenic lymphoma, phagocytosis of AMI-25 is markedly reduced, causing lymphomatous spleens to exhibit a higher-signal intensity postcontrast, compared with normal and enlarged (with benign disease) spleens. This permitted unambiguous identification of patients with diffuse infiltration of the spleen by lymphoma in this limited clinical trial.

Ultrasmall Superparamagnetic Iron Oxide Particles

Ultrasmall superparamagnetic iron oxide particles (USPIOs, with 70% of the particles smaller than 10 nm) have a prolonged blood half-life compared with

AMI-25 (81 versus 6 minutes in rats) and demonstrate transmigration through the capillary wall.[91] Potential applications include imaging of the bone marrow and lymphatic system, use as a long half-life perfusion agent for the brain or heart, and binding to carrier molecules for receptor-specific targeting. Animal experimentation in rats and rabbits has confirmed the potential for bone marrow imaging, with enhanced detection and differentiation of small tumor foci within the marrow.[93] Imaging of an animal model of nodal metastases has confirmed that tumor-bearing nodes can be differentiated from normal nodes by their lack of change in signal intensity following USPIO administration.[94] In normal animals, the maximum decrease in lymph node relaxation times was observed within 24 to 48 hours after contrast administration.

Ultrasmall Iron Oxide Particles Targeted to Asialoglycoprotein Receptors

Specific targeting of ultrasmall iron oxide particles to asialoglycoprotein receptors has been accomplished by coupling galactose terminals in the form of arabinogalactan to these particles.[95] Ultrasmall iron oxide particles targeted to asialoglycoprotein receptors (AG-USPIO) selectively accumulate in the liver.[96] Specificity for asialoglycoprotein (ASG) receptors has been confirmed by incubation experiments with and without blocking agents. In vivo on MRI, following contrast administration, there is a decrease in the signal intensity of normal hepatic tissue. This decrease is larger than that observed with conventional iron oxides at equivalent doses. Improved tumor–liver contrast has been demonstrated in animals following AG-USPIO administration.[97] This agent offers the potential both for markedly reduced dosage, compared with compounds such as AMI-25, as well as differentiation between benign (ASG-positive) and malignant (ASG-negative) hepatocellular tumors. Animal experiments also suggest that cellular hepatic abnormalities, such as that caused by fat replacement, hepatitis, or cirrhosis, can be detected and quantitated.[98]

HS

The HS MR agent (Advanced Magnetics Inc., Cambridge, Massachusetts) is similar in principle to AG-USPIO. It is an arabinogalactan-coated superparamagnetic iron oxide colloid that is removed from blood by the asialoglycoprotein receptor of hepatocytes. Like AG-USPIO, "the HS MR agent offers the prospect of visualizing the functional anatomy of noncancerous liver disease, as well as enhancing the contrast between tumor and normal tissue."[99] The optimum dose of Fe is estimated to be 7.5–10 μmol/kg, with an LD_{50} of ≥1800 μmol/kg.

ORAL CONTRAST MEDIA

Targeting of the gastrointestinal (GI) tract has been achieved by administration of oral contrast agents. Opacification of the gastrointestinal tract is important for enhanced discrimination of the gut from other organs and from pathologic lesions.[100] Two basic classes of these agents now exist for MRI: those that cause an increase in signal intensity (positive contrast agents), and those that cause a decrease in signal intensity (negative contrast agents). Gadopentetate dimeglumine serves as a prototype for the first class of agents, and superparamagnetic iron oxides for the second. Positive enhancement can lead to image degradation by motion artifacts from bowel peristalsis, a problem not encountered with negative agents. However, delineation of the bowel wall itself is best accomplished with positive agents. In addition to the substances described subsequently, limited investigation has been performed with magnetite albumin microspheres (MAM)[101] and various perfluorochemicals,[102] both of which create a signal void within the bowel. Infant-feeding formula is also known to be of high-signal intensity on T1- and T2-weighted imaging, providing for visualization of the gastrointestinal tract on MRI in newborns.[103] High-density barium sulfate suspensions behave as a negative oral contrast agent on both T1- and T2-weighted studies, with reports[104,105] advocating use as an interim solution before approval of agents specifically designed for MRI.

Gadopentetate Dimeglumine

Gadopentetate dimeglumine (Schering AG, Berlin, Germany), is in clinical trials in Europe[106] as a potential oral contrast agent, and clinical trials in the United States are anticipated in the near future. The formulation administered in Europe was 1.0 mmol/L gadopentetate dimeglumine mixed with 15 g mannitol per liter in water, and it was given in a dose of 10 mL/kg of body weight (the effective dose of gadopentetate dimeglumine is 0.01 mmol/kg). The mannitol has been added to give a more homogeneous opacification of bowel.

Pelvic and lower abdominal MRI is hampered by peristaltic motion, particularly when the bowel contents are high in signal intensity, as with oral preparations of gadopentetate dimeglumine. This problem can be resolved, in part, by the use of short repetition time (TR) sequences run with multiple acquisitions. Peristalsis can also be minimized with an injection of a hypotonic agent, such as glucagon. As fast-scan techniques become more common (such as those employed for breathhold imaging), problems related to artifacts from bowel peristalsis should diminish in severity.

dimeglumine yields clear distinction of abdominal bowel loops from intra-abdominal masses. Pathologic thickening of the bowel wall can also be identified. On T1-weighted images without oral contrast, the bowel and its liquid contents are isointense with soft tissue and muscle. After gadopentetate dimeglumine ingestion, the bowel contents are homogeneously high-signal intensity, differentiated from fecal material with intermediate-signal intensity and gas or air with low-signal intensity. In initial patient research, 19 of 32 studies showed improved delineation of abdominal abnormalities following oral gadopentetate dimeglumine administration.[107] Diarrhea was noted in some patients, presumably caused by the mannitol included in the oral preparation. In a subsequent larger series of 150 examinations, abdominal distension (by gas) and diarrhea were noted in 25% of patients within 24 hours of oral contrast administration.[108] T1-weighted images appear best for contrast delineation. Signal intensity measurements taken before and several hours after contrast administration suggest that gadopentetate dimeglumine is not absorbed in large amounts by the gastrointestinal tract.

It has been suggested on the basis of initial unenhanced MRI studies that improved visualization and delineation of the pancreas would require the use of an oral contrast agent.[109] In a subsequent series of 52 patients studied both before and after oral administration of gadopentetate dimeglumine, improved visualization of the pancreatic head, body, and tail was observed on enhanced scans in 15, 14, and 7 of 27 normal patients and 17, 8, and 6 of 25 patients with pancreatic disease.[110] Improved delineation was noted specifically of pancreatic pseudocysts and bowel wall invasion. Applications in the pelvis have also been described. In an initial study of 18 patients with pelvic tumors, improved delineation between tumor and intestine was demonstrated in 54% following oral contrast administration.[111]

Gadoterate Meglumine

Initial evaluation is in progress for an oral preparation of gadoterate meglumine.[112] Twenty-nine patients were studied after ingestion of 1000 mL of a 10% glucose solution containing 4 mL of gadoterate meglumine.

Paramagnetic Oil Emulsions

The combination of a paramagnetic agent, such as gadopentetate dimeglumine or ferric ammonium citrate, with an oil emulsion can serve as an effective oral contrast agent with high patient acceptance.[113] Various combinations with corn oil, olive oil, peanut oil, ice cream, and milk have been evaluated.

Oral Magnetic Particles

Superparamagnetic iron oxide particles are also being employed as oral contrast agents for the gastrointestinal tract on MRI. As previously noted, the use of a positive paramagnetic contrast medium, such as one of the gadolinium-based agents, produces high-signal intensity within the bowel, which can cause motion-related image degradation because of peristalsis. Oral magnetic particles (OMP, Nycomed AS, Oslo, Norway) act as negative contrast agents and, hence, do not cause motion-related image degradation (the degree of motion-related artifacts is proportional to the signal intensity of the structure from which they emanate). Oral magnetic particles and a related agent for intravenous administration, IMP, have been evaluated in vitro for their imaging characteristics.[114] The OMP agent is not biodegradable and, therefore, not absorbed from the digestive tract after ingestion.[115–117] Spheres (monodisperse polymer particles) measuring 3 to 4 μm in diameter are prepared in a liquid solution that the patient drinks before imaging. The active component of the contrast agent consists of crystalline (ferrite-type) magnetic iron oxide (50 nm in diameter), which is coated on the carrier matrix. The iron content is 20% to 27% by weight. Iron particles cause local magnetic field inhomogeneities, with the bowel thus appearing as low-signal intensity, or black, on MR scans, permitting delineation of abnormality within and adjacent to the gastrointestinal tract. Two concentrations of OMP have been used clinically, 0.25 and 0.5 g/L, with the total administered volume being 800 mL. T1-, T2-, and proton-density–weighted spin echo sequences

have been applied at different field strengths from 0.02 to 1.5 T. Sufficient or excellent contrast effect (signal void) has been demonstrated on all applied sequences. The contrast medium is typically evenly distributed and gives good contrast enhancement in both the upper and lower abdomen. Even distribution of the contrast medium has been achieved by formulation of OMP with starch and cellulose. Thirty-one male patients with testicular cancer, and 31 female patients with lower abdominal and pelvic disease, have been examined in two Phase II clinical trials.[118] In the second trial, the diagnostic information available from postcontrast scans was greater than that from precontrast scans in 16 patients (52%) (Fig. 5–15). Uncommon side effects included nausea and vomiting. A change in bowel habits during the week following examination (both loose stools and constipation) was reported by 29 patients. Now in Phase III clinical trials, the agent has been well accepted by patients,[119] with no serious side effects reported (personal communication, Nycomed AS Imaging, Oslo, Norway). Utility has also been shown in imaging of patients with acute pancreatitis and lymphoma. Approximately 450 patients have now been studied.

AMI-121

An oral formulation of superparamagnetic iron oxide particles has been prepared by Advanced Magnetics Inc: AMI-121 (personal communication, Advanced Magnetics Inc, Cambridge, Massachusetts). AMI-121 is a colloidal preparation of nonabsorbable, superparamagnetic iron oxide particles. The superparamagnetic characteristics[120] of this material, like OMP, create local inhomogeneities in the MR magnetic field that markedly reduce the T2 relaxation time in the region of the imaging agent. After oral administration of the agent and transit of AMI-121 into the bowel, the lumen of the gastrointestinal tract appears dark on images (Fig. 5–16). The agent is not absorbed and is excreted within 6 to 24 hours after administration (depending upon bowel transit time). AMI-121 has completed Phase III clinical trials.

SUMMARY

Since the development of gadopentetate dimeglumine, many additional MRI contrast agents have been formulated, providing the potential for further improvements in pathologic diagnosis. The range of possible applications for MRI contrast media has also been expanded by the development of new MRI hardware and software, including dynamic imaging and MR angiography. Owing to these developments, cardiac and abdominal imaging are likely to be employed clinically on a more routine

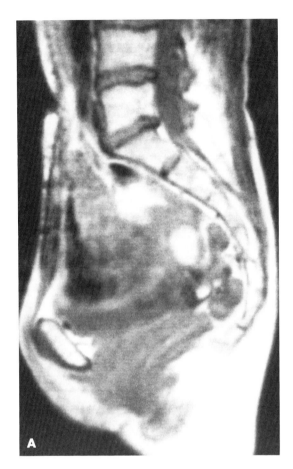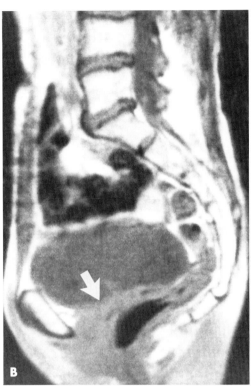

FIGURE 5-15 Oral magnetic particles: colon carcinoma. T1-weighted (TR/TE = 450/20) sagittal images **(A)** before and **(B)** after oral magnetic particle (OMP) administration. On the postcontrast image, low-signal intensity is noted identifying the lumen of small bowel, sigmoid colon, and rectum. A large soft-tissue mass (*arrow,* **B**) is best recognized, surrounding the rectosigmoid, on the postcontrast section. (Courtesy of Professor Peter A. Rinck, MR center, Trondheim, Norway)

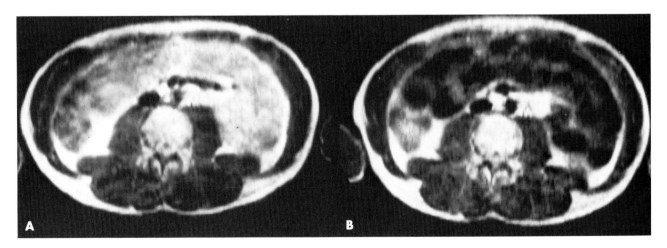

FIGURE 5-16 AMI-121: normal volunteer. T2-weighted (TR/TE = 1500/40) images **(A)** pre- and **(B)** post-AMI-121 ingestion (Fe, 175 µg/mL). Uniform intraluminal darkening clearly outlines the extent of the bowel on the postcontrast image. (Courtesy of Advanced Magnetics Inc, Cambridge, Massachusetts)

Table 5–2 **Contrast Media for MRI in Clinical Trials or Approved for Clinical Use**

AGENT	LD$_{50}$*	RECOMMENDED DOSE	$t_{1/2}$ (ELIMINATION)	DISTRIBUTION	OSMOLALITY (mOsm/kg)
Gd-DTPA (Magnevist)	10	0.1 mmol/kg	96 min	ECF	1960[1]
Gd-DOTA (Dotarem)	18[1]	0.1 mmol/kg	90 min[2]	ECF	1400[3]
Gd-HP-DO3A (ProHance)	12[4]	0.1 mmol/kg	94 min†	ECF	630†
GD-DTPA-BMA (Omniscan)	14§	0.1 mmol/kg	78 min§	ECF	789§
Gd-BOPTA	5.8[64]‖	250 μmol/kg	N/A	ECF (partial biliary excretion)	~750[64]
Mn-DPDP	3‡‖	10 μmol/kg	N/A	Extracellular and intracellular	1200§
AMI-25	N/A	20 μmolFe/kg	N/A	RE system	N/A
Gd-DTPA (oral formulation)	N/A	10 mL/kg (1.0 mM concentration)	N/A	GI tract	N/A
Gd-DOTA (oral formulation)	N/A	1000 mL	N/A	GI tract	N/A
Oral magnetic particles	N/A	800 mL (0.5 g/L concentration)	N/A	GI tract	N/A
AMI-121	N/A	N/A	N/A	GI tract	N/A

Abbreviations: N/A, not available; ECF, extracellular fluid.
*mmol/kg in rats (unless otherwise noted).
†Personal communication, Bristol-Myers-Squibb Diagnostics, New Brunswick, New Jersey.
‡Personal communication, Nycomed AS Imaging, Oslo, Norway.
§Personal communication, Salutar Inc., Sunnyvale, California.
‖ mmol/kg in mice.

basis in the future, placing additional demands upon, and opening further avenues of application for, contrast media. In addition to the agents described in this chapter, many other compounds are currently being formulated and tested in research laboratories at both academic sites and in industry.

Two extracellular gadolinium chelates (gadopentetate dimeglumine and gadoterate meglumine), with predominant renal excretion, are currently approved in the world for use in patients. Approval of additional agents in this specific class is anticipated within the next year, with the potential for high dose (0.2–0.3 mmol/kg) contrast use demonstrated with gadoteridol. It is likely that agents targeted to the liver will also be approved for clinical use, although these are not as far along in clinical evaluation. It is difficult to predict which type of agent will eventually be used clinically in the liver. Extracellular gadolinium chelates have been employed successfully with breathhold dynamic imaging; however, other approaches, including particulate substances (for example, AG-USPIO) and extracellular agents with hepatobiliary uptake, appear promising. Clinical approval of both positive and negative oral contrast media is anticipated as well in the future. The various agents, both intravenous and oral, that have received clinical attention are listed in Table 5–2, together with pertinent physicochemical properties, as compiled from the scientific literature. As with magnetic resonance imaging itself, development of contrast media has far exceeded initial expectations and will continue to play a dominant role in this exciting dynamic field.[121]

REFERENCES

1. Weinmann HJ, Press WR, Gries H. Tolerance of extracellular contrast agents for MRI [abstract]. In: Contrast media research 1989. Sydney and Hamilton Island, Australia: 1989: MR9.
2. Doucet D, Meyer D, Bonnemain B, et al. Gd-DOTA. In: Runge V, ed. Enhanced magnetic resonance imaging. St Louis: CV Mosby, 1989:87–104.
3. Schaeffer M, Meyer D, Doucet D. Advances in macrocyclic gadolinium complexes as MRI contrast agents. In: Proceedings of the European Congress on NMR in Medicine and Biology 1990. Strasbourg, France.
4. Tweedle M, Chang C, Dischino D, et al. Gadolinium chelates for cerebral and myocardial imaging [abstract]. In: Contrast media research 1989. Sydney and Hamilton Island, Australia: 1989: MR12.
5. Runge VM, Carollo BR, Wolf CR, et al. Gd-DTPA: a review of clinical indications in central nervous system magnetic resonance imaging. Radiographics 1989;9:929–958.
6. Russell EJ, Schiable TF, Dillon W, et al. Multicenter double-blind placebo-controlled study of gadopentetate dimeglumine as an MR contrast agent: evaluation in patients with cerebral lesions. AJR 1989;152:813–823.
7. Nelson KL, Runge VM. Thoracic spine. In: Runge VM, ed. Clinical magnetic resonance imaging. Philadelphia: JB Lippincott, 1990;233–253.
8. Ross JS, Modic MT, Masaryk TJ, et al. Assessment of extradural degenerative disease with Gd DTPA-enhanced MR imaging: correlation with surgical and pathologic findings. AJR 1990; 154:151–157.
9. Parizel PM, Baleriaux D, Rodesh G, et al. Gd-DTPA-enhanced MR imaging of spinal tumors. AJR 1989;152:1087–1096.
10. Bloem JL, Reiser MF, Vanel D. Magnetic resonance contrast agents in the evaluation of the musculoskeletal system. Magn Reson Q 1990;6:136–163.
11. Erlemann R, Reiser M, Peters P, et al. Musculoskeletal neoplasms: static and dynamic Gd DTPA-enhanced MR imaging. Radiology 1989;17:767–773.

12. Bjorkengren AG, Geborek P, Rydholm U, et al. MR imaging of the knee in acute rheumatoid arthritis: synovial uptake of gadolinium-DOTA. AJR 1990;155:329–332.

13. Busch JJ, Nelson JF, Cadena G. MR shoulder arthrography: 3D FISP imaging of the labrum [abstract]. J Magn Reson Imaging 1991;1:152.

14. Van-Rossum AC, Visser FC, Eenige MJ, et al. Value of gadolinium-diethylenetriamine pentaacetic acid dynamics in magnetic resonance imaging of acute myocardial infarction with occluded and reperfused coronary arteries after thrombolysis. Am J Cardiol 1990;65:845–851.

15. Hamm B, Laniado M, Saini S. Contrast-enhanced magnetic resonance imaging of the abdomen and pelvis. Magn Reson Q 1990;6:108–135.

16. Edelman RR, Siegel JB, Singer A, et al. Dynamic MR imaging of the liver with Gd-DTPA: initial clinical results. AJR 1989;153:1213–1219.

17. Creasy JL, Price RR, Presbey T, et al. Gadolinium-enhanced MR angiography. Radiology 1990;175:280–283.

18. Niendorf HP, Laniado M, Semmler W, et al. Dose administration of gadolinium DTPA in MR imaging of intracranial tumors. AJNR 1987;8:803–815.

19. Hamm B. Liver. In: Runge VM, ed. Enhanced magnetic resonance imaging. St Louis: CV Mosby, 1989:244–267.

20. Heywang SH, Worl A, Pruss E, et al. MR imaging of the breast with Gd DTPA: use and limitations. Radiology 1989;171:95–103.

21. de Roos A, Matheijssen NAA, Doornbos J, et al. Myocardial infarct size after reperfusion therapy: assessment with Gd DTPA enhanced MR imaging. Radiology 1990;176:517–521.

22. Schubeus P, Schoerner W. Dosing of Gd DTPA in MR imaging of intracranial tumors. In: Workshop on contrast enhanced magnetic resonance imaging. Napa, Calif: Society of Magnetic Resonance in Medicine, 1991:109–123.

23. Runge VM, Kirsch JE, Burke V, et al. High dose application of gadoteridol in brain MRI. (In press).

24. Rosen BR, Belliveau JW, Vevea JM, et al. Perfusion imaging with NMR contrast agents. Magn Reson Med 1990;14:249–265.

25. Edelman RR, Mattle HP, Atkinson DJ, et al. Cerebral blood flow: assessment with dynamic contrast enhanced T2* weighted MR imaging at 1.5 T. Radiology 1990;176:211–220.

26. Hamm B, Fischer E, Taupitz M. Differentiation of hepatic hemangiomas from metastases by dynamic contrast-enhanced MR imaging. J Comput Assist Tomogr 1990;14:205–216.

27. Cuenod CA, Bellin MF, Bousquet JC, et al. MRI of liver tumors using gadolinium DOTA: prospective study comparing spin echo long TR-TE sequence and CT. Magn Reson Imaging 1991;9:235–245.

28. Marchal G, Demaerel P, Decrop E, et al. Gadolinium-DOTA enhanced fast imaging of liver tumors at 1.5 T. J Comput Assist Tomogr 1990;14:217–222.

29. Mirowitz SA, Lee JK, Gutierrez E, et al. Dynamic gadolinium enhanced rapid acquisition spin echo MR imaging of the liver. Radiology 1991;179:371–376.

30. Yoshida H, Itai Y, Ohtomo K, et al. Small hepatocellular carcinoma and cavernous hemangioma: differentiation with dynamic FLASH MR imaging with Gd DTPA. Radiology 1989;171:339–342.

31. Runge VM, Kirsch JE, Thomas GS. High dose applications of gadolinium chelates in magnetic resonance imaging. In: Workshop on contrast enhanced magnetic resonance imaging. Napa, Calif: Society of Magnetic Resonance in Medicine, 1991:300–306.

32. McClennan BL. Ionic and nonionic iodinated contrast media: evolution and strategies for use. AJR 1990;155:255–263.

33. Cacheris WP, Quay SC, Rocklage SM. The relationship between thermodynamics and the toxicity of gadolinium complexes. Magn Reson Imaging 1990;8:467–481.

34. Rocklage SM. Metal ion release from paramagnetic chelates: what is tolerable? In: Workshop on contrast enhanced magnetic resonance imaging. Napa, Calif: Society of Magnetic Resonance in Medicine, 1991: 56–69.

35. Gennaro MC, Aime S, Santucci E, et al. Complexes of diethylenetriaminepentaacetic acid as contrast agents in NMR image. Computer simulation of equilibria in human blood plasma. Anal Chim Acta 1990;233:85–100.

36. Sherry AD. Lanthanide chelates as magnetic resonance imaging contrast agents. J Less Common Metals 1989;149:133–141.

37. Goldstein HA, Kashanian FK, Blumetti RF, et al. Safety assessment of gadopentetate dimeglumine in US clinical trials. Radiology 1990;174:17–23.

38. Bydder GM. Clinical use of contrast media in magnetic resonance imaging. Br J Hosp Med 1990;43:149–152.

39. Powers TA, Partain CL, Kessler RM, et al. Central nervous lesions in pediatric patients: Gd-DTPA-enhanced MR imaging. Radiology 1988;169:723–726.

40. Runge VM, Gelblum DY. The role of gadolinium-diethylenetriaminepentaacetic acid in the evaluation of the central nervous system. Magn Reson Q 1990;6:85–107.

41. Runge VM. Contrast media. In: Runge VM, ed. Clinical magnetic resonance imaging. Philadelphia: JB Lippincott, 1990:517–548.

42. Neindorf HP, Haustein J, Alhassan A, Clauss W. Safety of gadolinium DTPA: extended clinical experience. In: Workshop on contrast enhanced magnetic resonance imaging. Napa, Calif: Society of Magnetic Resonance in Medicine, 1991: 70–79.

43. Niendorf HP, Seifert W. Serum iron and serum bilirubin after administration of Gd DTPA dimeglumine: a pharmacologic study in healthy volunteers. Invest Radiol 1988;23(suppl 1):S275–S280.

44. Schmeidl U, Maravilla R, Gerlach R, Dowling CA. Excretion of gadopentetate dimeglumine in human breast milk. AJR 1990; 154:1305–1306.

45. Wolf GL. Current status of MR imaging contrast agents: special report. Radiology 1989;172:709–710.

46. Kanal E, Applegate GR, Gillen CP. Review of adverse reactions, including anaphylaxis, in 4260 intravenous bolus injections [abstract]. Radiology 1990;177(P):159.

47. Weiss KL. Severe anaphylactoid reaction after IV Gd-DTPA. Magn Reson Imaging 1990;8:817–818.

48. Meyer D, Schaefer M, Doucet D. Advances in macrocyclic gadolinium complexes as magnetic resonance imaging contrast agents. Invest Radiol 1990;25:S53–S55.

49. Parizel PM, Degryse HR, Gheuens J, et al. Gadolinium DOTA enhanced MR imaging of intracranial lesions. J Comput Assist Tomogr 1989;13:378–385.

50. Jau P, Bonnet JL, Joly P, et al. Acute myocardial infarction evaluation by magnetic resonance imaging with injection of gadolinium DOTA. Arch Mal Coeur 1991;84:195–200.

51. Neiss AC, Le Mignon MM, Vitry A, Caille JM. Efficacy and tolerability of Gd-DOTA in a European multicentre survey. (submitted for publication).

52. Le Mignon MM, Chambon C, Warrington S, et al. Gd-DOTA: pharmacokinetics and tolerability after intravenous injection into healthy volunteers. Invest Radiol 1990;25:933–937.

53. Dischino DD, Delaney EJ, Emswiler JE, et al. Synthesis of non-ionic gadolinium chelates useful as contrast agents for magnetic resonance imaging. 1, 4, 7-Tris(Carboxymethyl)-10-substituted-1, 4, 7, 10-tetraazacyclododecanes and their corresponding gadolinium chelates. Inorg Chem 1991; (in press).

54. Chang CA, Kumar K, Garrison JM, et al. Physicochemical properties of Gd (HP-DO3A)—a nonionic macrocyclic magnetic resonance imaging contrast agent [abstract]. Soc Magn Reson Med 1990:729.

55. Runge V, Gelblum D, Pacetti M, et al. Gd HP-DO3A in clinical MR of the brain. Radiology 1990;177:393–400.

56. Tweedle MF. Work in progress toward nonionic macrocyclic gadolinium (III) complexes. In: Rinck PA, ed. Contrast and contrast agents in magnetic resonance imaging, European workshop on magnetic resonance in medicine, 1989:65–73.

57. Tweedle MF, Hagan JJ, Kumar K, et al. Reaction of gadolinium chelates with endogenously available ions. Magn Reson Imaging 1991; (in press).

58. Runge VM, Bradley WG, Brant-Zawadzki MN, et al. Clinical safety and efficacy of gadoteridol (Gd HP-DO3A)—a study of 411 patients with suspected intracranial and spinal pathology. Radiology 1991; (in press)

59. Greco A, McNamara MT, Lanthiez P, et al. Gadodiamide injection: nonionic gadolinium chelate for MR imaging of the brain and spine—phase II-III clinical trial. Radiology 1990;176:451–456.

60. Aisen AM, Kaplan G, Aravapalli SR. A clinical trial of gadolinium-DTPA-bis-(methylamide) [abstract]. Magn Reson Imaging 1990;8(S1):46.

61. Weinmann HJ, Press WR, Gries H. Tolerance of extracellular contrast agents for magnetic resonance imaging. Invest Radiol 1990;25:S49–S50.

62. Meyer D, Schaefer M, Doucet D. Advances in macrocyclic imaging. Society of Magnetic Resonance in Medicine, 1991:80–87. Invest Radiol 1990;25:S53–S55.

63. Schaefer M, Meyer D, Beaute S, Doucet D. A new macrocyclic MRI contrast agent: Gd MCTA complex. In: Workshop on contrast enhanced magnetic resonance imaging. Napa, Calif: Society of Magnetic Resonance in Medicine, 1991: 88–98.

64. Vittadine G, Felder E, Musu C, Tirone P. Preclinical profile of Gd BOPTA: a liver-specific MRI contrast agent. Invest Radiol 1990;25:S59–S60.

65. Cavagna F, Dapra M, Maggioni F, et al. Gd BOPTA/dimeglumine: experimental disease imaging. In: Workshop on contrast enhanced magnetic resonance imaging. Napa, Calif: Society of Magnetic Resonance in Medicine, 1991: 243–251.

66. Weinmann HJ, Schuhmann-Giampieri G, Schmitt-Willich H, et al. A new lipophilic gadolinium chelate as a tissue-specific contrast media for MRI. In: Workshop on contrast enhanced magnetic resonance imaging. Society of Magnetic Resonance in Medicine, 1991:80–87.

67. Hahn PF, Stark DD, Weissleder R, et al. Clinical applications of superparamagnetic iron oxide to MR imaging of tissue perfusion in vascular liver tumors. Radiology 1990;174:361–366.

68. Golman K, Klaveness J, Holtz E, et al. A magnetic resonance imaging contrast medium for the liver and bile. Invest Radiol 1988;23(S):243–245.

69. Unger E. Theoretical considerations for the design of targeted MR contrast agents [abstract]. Magn Reson Imaging 1990; 8(S1):41.

70. Saeed M, Wendland MF, Tomei E, et al. Demarcation of mycardial ischemia: magnetic susceptibility effect of contrast medium in MR imaging. Radiology 1989;173:763–767.

71. Moseley ME, Kucharczyk J, Mintorovitch J, et al. Diffusion weighted MR imaging of acute stroke: correlation with T2-weighted and magnetic susceptibility enhanced MR imaging in cats. AJNR 1990;11:423–429.

72. Elizondo G, Fretz CJ, Stark DD, et al. Preclinical evaluation of Mn DPDP: new paramagnetic hepatobiliary contrast agent for MR imaging. Radiology 1991;178:73–78.

73. Lim KO, Stark DD, Leese PT, et al. Hepatobiliary MR imaging: first human experience with MN DPDP. Radiology 1991;178:79–82.

74. Bernardino ME. Clinical hepatic imaging with paramagnetic positive enhancers. In: Workshop on contrast enhanced magnetic resonance imaging. Napa, Calif: Society of Magnetic Resonance in Medicine, 1991: 252–262.

75. Young SW, Bradley B, Muller HH, Rubin DL. Detection of hepatic malignancies using Mn-DPDP (Manganese dipyridoxal disphosphate) hepatobiliary MRI contrast agent. Magn Reson Imaging 1990;8:267–276.

76. Young SW, Simpson BB, Ratner AV, et al. MRI measurement of hepatocyte toxicity using a new MRI contrast agent manganese dipyridoxal diphosphate, a manganese/pyridoxal 5-phosate chelate. Magn Reson Med 1989;10:1–13.

77. Pomeroy OH, Wendland M, Wagner S, et al. Magnetic resonance imaging of acute myocardial ischemia using a manganese chelate, Mn-DPTP. Invest Radiol 1989;24:531–536.

78. Saeed M, Wagner S, Wendland MF, et al. Occlusive and reperfused myocardial infarcts: differentiation with Mn-DPDP enhanced MR imaging. Radiology 1989;172:59–64.

79. Shtern F, Garrido L, Compton C, et al. MR imaging of bloodborne liver metastases in mice: contrast enhancement with Fe EHPG. Radiology 1991;178:83–89.

80. Lauffer RB, Vincent AC, Padmanabhan S, et al. Hepatobiliary MR contrast agents: 5-substituted iron-EHPG derivatives. Magn Reson Med 1987;4:582–590.

81. Weissleder R. Target specific superparamagnetic MR contrast agents. In: Workshop on contrast enhanced magnetic resonance imaging. Napa, Calif: Society of Magnetic Resonance in Medicine, 1991: 47–54.

82. Cerdan S, Lotscher HR, Kunnecke B, Seelig J. Monoclonal antibody coated magnetite particles as contrast agents in magnetic resonance imaging of tumors. Magn Reson Med 1989; 12:151–163.

83. Stark DD, Weissleder R, Elizondo G, et al. Superparamagnetic iron oxide: clinical application as a contrast agent for MR imaging of the liver. Radiology 1988;168:297–301.

84. Weissleder R, Stark DD, Engelstad BL, et al. Superparamagnetic iron oxide: pharmacokinetics and toxicity. AJR 1989;152:167–73.

85. Clement O, Schouman-Claeys E, Frija G. Ferrite particles (AMI-25): influence of cirrhosis and chemotheraphy on MR imaging of hepatic metastasis [abstract]. In: Contrast media research 1989. Sydney and Hamilton Island, Australia. 1989: MR20.

86. Gundersen HG, Bach-Gansmo T, Holtz E, et al. Clinical usefulness of superparamagnetic contrast agents for MRI [abstract]. In: Contrast media research 1989. Sydney and Hamilton Island, Australia. 1989: MR23.

87. Clement O, Schouman-Claeys E, Frija G. Ferrite particles (AMI-25): influence of cirrhosis and chemotherapy on magnetic resonance imaging of metastasis. Invest Radiol 1990;25:S61–S62.

88. Stark DD, Weissleder R, Elizondo G, et al. Superparamagnetic iron oxide: clinical application as a contrast agent for MR imaging of the liver. Radiology 1988;168:297–301.

89. Hahn PF, Stark DD, Weissleder R, et al. Clinical application of superparamagnetic iron oxide to MR imaging of tissue perfusion in vascular liver tumors. Radiology 1990;174:361–366.

90. Weissleder R, Hahn PF, Stark DD, et al. Superparamagnetic iron oxide: enhanced detection of focal splenic tumors with MR imaging. Radiology 1988;169:399–403.

91. Weissleder R, Elizondo G, Stark DD, et al. The diagnosis of splenic lymphoma by MR imaging: value of superparamagnetic iron oxide. AJR 1989;152:175–180.

92. Weissleder R, Elizondo G, Wittenberg J, et al. Ultrasmall superparamagnetic iron oxide: characterization of a new class of contrast agents for MR imaging. Radiology 1990;175:489–493.

93. Seneterre E, Weissleder R, Jaramillo D, et al. Bone marrow: ultrasmall superparamagnetic iron oxide for MR imaging. Radiology 1991;179:529–533.

94. Weissleder R, Elizondo G, Wittenberg J, et al. Ultrasmall superparamagnetic iron oxide: an intravenous contrast agent for assessing lymph nodes with MR imaging. Radiology 1990; 175:494–498.

95. Weissleder R, Reimer P, Lee A, et al. MR receptor imaging: ultrasmall iron oxide particles targeted to asialoglycoprotein receptors [abstract]. Radiology 1990;177(P):110.

96. Weissleder R, Reimer P, Lee AS, et al. MR receptor imaging: ultrasmall iron oxide particles targeted to asialoglycoprotein receptors. AJR 1990;155:1161–1167.

97. Reimer P, Weissleder R, Lee AS, et al. Receptor imaging: application to MR imaging of liver cancer. Radiology 1990; 177:729–734.

98. Reimer P, Weissleder R, Lee AS, et al. Asialoglycoprotein receptor function in benign liver disease: evaluation with MR imaging. Radiology 1991;178:769–774.

99. Josephson L, Groman EV, Menz E, et al. A functionalized superparamagnetic iron oxide colloid as a receptor directed MR contrast agent. Magn Reson Imaging 1990;8:637–646.

100. Hamm B, Laniado M, Saini S. Contrast enhanced magnetic resonance imaging of the abdomen and pelvis. Magn Reson Q 1990;6:108–135.

101. Widder DJ, Edelman RR, Grief WI, Monda L. Magnetite albumin suspension: a superparamagnetic oral MR contrast agent. AJR 1987;149:839–843.

102. Mattrey RF, Hajek PC, Gylys-Morin VM, et al. Perfluorochemicals as gastrointestinal contrast agents for MR imaging: preliminary studies in rats and humans. AJR 1987; 148:1259–1263.

103. Gerscovich EO, McGahan JP, Buonocore MH, et al. The rediscovery of infant feeding formula with magnetic resonance imaging. Pediatr Radiol 1990;20:147–151.

104. King CPL, Tart RP, Fitzsimmons JR, et al. Barium sulfate suspension as a negative oral MRI contrast agent: in vitro and human optimization studies. Magn Reson Imaging 1991;9:141–150.

105. Marti-Bonmati L, Vilar J, Paniagua JC, Talens A. High density barium sulphate as an MRI oral contrast. Magn Reson Imaging 1991;9:259–261.

106. Laniado M, Kornmesser W, Hamm B, et al. MR imaging of the gastrointestinal tract: value of Gd-DTPA. AJR 1988;150:817–821.

107. Claussen C, Kornmesser W, Laniado M, et al. Oral contrast media for magnetic resonance tomography of the abdomen: III. initial patient research with gadolinium DTPA. ROFO 1988;148:683–689.

108. Krahe T, Dolken W, Lackner K, et al. Gadolinium DTPA as an oral contrast medium for MR tomography of the abdomen. ROFO 1990;153:167–173.

109. Piccirillo M, Bourque A, McCarthy S, Lange R. High field imaging of the normal pancreas. Magn Reson Imaging 1989;7:457–461.

110. Neumann K, Kaminsky S, Gogoll M, et al. Gadolinium DTPA as an oral contrast medium for magnetic resonance tomography of the pancreas. ROFO 1991;154:262–268.

111. Hotzinger H, Salbeck R, Toedt C, Beyer HK. Initial experience with the use of oral gadolinium DTPA in nuclear magnetic resonance tomography of the pelvis. Digitale Bilddiagn 1990; 10:42–45.

112. Miaux Y, Frija J, Dubourdieux C, et al. Interet du DOTA-gadolinium oral dans l'IRM de l'abdomen [abstract]. European Research Congress on Contrast Products, Lyon, March 1991.

113. Li KC, Ang PG, Tart RP, et al. Paramagnetic oil emulsions as oral magnetic resonance imaging contrast agents. Magn Reson Imaging 1990;8:589–598.

114. Ericsson A, Lonnemark M, Hemmingsson A, Bach-Gansmo T. Effect of superparamagnetic particles in agarose gels. A magnetic resonance imaging study. Acta Radiol 1991;32:74–78.

115. Kean D, Best J, Turnbull L, et al. Oral magnetic particles: a new contrast agent for abdominal MR imaging [abstract]. Soc Magn Reson Med 1989:790.

116. Rinck PA, Smevik O, Nilsen G, et al. Abdominal and pelvic contrast enhancement using oral magnetic particles [abstract]. Soc Magn Reson Med, 1989:354.

117. Lonnemark M, Hemmingsson A, Bach Gansmo T, et al. Effect of superparamagnetic particles as oral medium at magnetic resonance imaging. A phase I clinical study. Acta Radiol 1989;30:193–196.

118. Rinck PA, Smevik O, Nilsen G, et al. Oral magnetic particles in MR imaging of the abdomen and pelvis. Radiology 1991;178:775–779.

119. Lonnemark M, Hemmingsson A, Bach-Gansmo T, et al. Effect of superparamagnetic particles as oral contrast medium at magnetic resonance imaging. A phase I clinical study. Acta Radiol 1989;30:193–196.

120. Erquiaga E, Ros PR, Torres GM, et al. Oral superparamagnetic iron oxide: use in pancreatic MR imaging [abstract]. Radiology 1990;177:377.

121. Saini S, Modic MT, Hamm B, Hahn PF. Advances in contrast-enhanced MR imaging. AJR 1991;156:235–254.

Appendix

Brain

	TR (ms)	TE (ms)	SLICE THICKNESS	INTERSLICE GAP (%)	FOV (cm)	EXCITATIONS	MATRIX[†]	SCAN TIME (min : s)
Screening Examination								
Precontrast								
1. Sagittal scout	500	10	5	30	23	1	192*256	1:40
2. Axial T2	2500	45,90[‡]	7	30	23	1	256*256	10:44
3. Axial T1	600	22[‡]	7	30	23	2	256*256	5:11
Postcontrast								
4. Axial T1	(Use parameters as above)							
5. Coronal T1	(Optional-use parameters as defined for sagittal precontrast scan)							
6. Sagittal T1	(Optional-use parameters as defined for precontrast scan)							
Posterior Fossa (thin section)								
Precontrast								
1. Sagittal scout	500	10	5	30	23	1	192*256	1:40
2. Axial T2	3000	45,90[‡]	3	30	25	1	220*256	11:05
3. Axial T1	600	10	3	30	25	2	220*256	4:27
4. Coronal T1	600	10	3	30	25	2	220*256	4:27
Postcontrast								
5. Axial T1	(Use parameters as defined for precontrast scan)							
6. Coronal T1	(Use parameters as defined for precontrast scan)							
Sella								
Precontrast								
1. Sagittal T1	500	15	3	30	22	3	256*256	6:28
2. Coronal T2	3000	45,90[‡]	3	30	25	1	220*256	11:05
3. Coronal T1	500	22[‡]	3	30	22	3	256*256	6:28
Postcontrast								
4. Coronal T1	(Use parameters as above)							
5. Sagittal T1	(Use parameters as defined for precontrast scan)							

†Phase encoding * readout gradient steps.
‡Sequence employs gradient moment refocusing (GMR).

Spine*

	TR (ms)	TE (ms)	SLICE THICKNESS	INTERSLICE GAP (%)	FOV (cm)	EXCITATIONS	MATRIX†	SCAN TIME (min : s)
Cervical								
Precontrast								
1. Sagittal T1	450	10	3	30	25	3	256*256	5:49
2. Sagittal T2	>2300	45,90‡	3	30	30	1	256*256	>9:56§
3. Sagittal FLASH‖, FA = 10⁰	300	10‡	4	20	25	1	192*256	1:00
4. Axial FISP, FA = 20⁰	250	12‡	4	20	25	4	256*256	4:19
5. Axial T1	470	10	3	30	25	2	256*256	4:04
Postcontrast								
6. Axial T1	(Use parameters as above)							
7. Sagittal T1	(Use parameters as defined for precontrast scan)							
Thoracic								
Precontrast								
1. Sagittal T1	450	10	3	30	25	2	256*256	3:54
2. Sagittal T2	>2300	45,90‡	3	30	30	1	256*256	>9:56§
3. Axial T1	705	10	3	30	25	2	256*256	6:05
Postcontrast								
4. Axial T1	(Use parameters as above)							
5. Sagittal T1	(Use parameters as defined for precontrast scan)							
Lumbar								
Precontrast								
1. Sagittal T1	450	10	4	30	25	3	256*256	5:49
2. Sagittal T2	3000	30,80‡	4	30	28	1	256*256	12:53
3. Axial T1	650	10	3	30	25	3	256*256	8:23
Postcontrast								
4. Axial T1	(Use parameters as above)							
5. Sagittal T1	(Use parameters as defined for precontrast scan)							

*A coronal presaturation slab should be employed on all spine examinations to diminish motion-related artifacts.
†Phase encoding * readout gradient steps.
‡Sequence employs gradient moment refocusing (GMR).
§ECG gated.
‖ Quick T2*-weighted scan.

Liver

	TR (ms)	TE (ms)	SLICE THICKNESS	INTERSLICE GAP (%)	FOV (cm)	EXCITATIONS	MATRIX†	SCAN TIME (min : s)
Precontrast								
1. Axial T2	2500	45,90‡	10	30	40	2	128*256	10:44
2. Axial T1	300	10	10	30	40	6	128*256	3:54
3. Axial T1 breathhold	260	10	10	30	40	1	64*256§	0:12
Postcontrast								
4. Axial T1 breathhold‖	(Use parameters as above)							
5. Axial T1	(Use parameters as defined for precontrast scan)							

†Phase encoding * readout gradient steps.
‡Sequence employs gradient moment refocusing (GMR).
§Rectangular field of view, half-Fourier acquisition. Spatial resolution is equivalent to a 128*256 matrix.
‖ This scan should be obtained as a dynamic study 1 to 2 minutes following bolus IV gadolinium chelate administration.

Index

The letter *f* after a page number indicates a figure; *t* following a page number indicates tabular material. Mathematical symbols are grouped at the beginning of the index.

Symbols

μ (mass absorption coefficient), 2

ρ (spin density), 3

τ^* (resonance correlation time), 10–11, 11f

τ_C. *See* Correlation times

τ_D (translational diffusion motion), 8

τ_e (spin-exchange correlation time), 10

τ_M (water molecule residence in bound state), 7–8

τ_R (tumbling time), 9–10

τ_S (electron-spin relaxation time), 9–10, 12–14, 13f–14f

τ_V (correlation time of frequency-dependent quantum mechanical spin state), 12

χ. *See* Susceptibility

d (distance between metal complex and water molecule), 8

D (diffusion coefficient), 5

[*M*] (paramagnetic concentration), 6–7

q (water molecules bound to paramagnetic ion), 8–9

R (relaxivity), 10

S (total electron spin of ion), 9

Z (atomic number), 2

A

Abdominal imaging, bowel labeling in, 120

Abscess
  of brain, 37, 48f–49f
  of spine, 101, 105f

Acoustic neuroma, 25, 31f–32f, 133f

Adenoma
  adrenal, 122
  pituitary, 33–34, 45f

Adrenal tumors, 121–122, 121f

AMI-25 contrast agent, 141–142, 142f, 146t

AMI-121 contrast agent, 144, 145f, 146t

Angioma, of brain, 52, 58, 59f

Annulus fibrosis
  degeneration of, 81–82
  imaging of, 70f–71f, 72, 76

Antibody-labeled iron oxide particles, 141

Arachnoid adhesions, spinal, 106f, 107

Arachnoiditis, spinal, 107

Arterial portography, 120

Arteriovenous malformations
  of brain, 52, 58, 59f
  of spinal cord, 79, 101, 104f, 108, 109f

Artifacts, in spinal imaging, 78–81

Asialoglycoprotein receptors, iron oxide particles targeted to, 141–143

Aspergillosis, spinal, 106f

Astrocytoma

Astrocytoma
  of brain, 27, 29, 33f, 36f
  of spine, 78, 90, 92, 93f, 138f

Atomic number, contrast and, 2

B

Barium sulfate, as contrast agent, 143

Basivertebral venous plexus, imaging of, 72, 73f, 75f–76f

Benzyloxymethyl-substituted diethylene-triamine pentaacetic acid, as gadolinium ligand, 130f, 138

Bilirubin levels, gadopentetate dimeglumine effects on, 132

Bladder tumors, 122

Blood-brain barrier disruption
  in infarction, 50, 55f–58f
  visualization of, 27, 29, 34f, 66f

Body imaging, 113–125
  in adrenal mass, 121–122, 121f
  in bowel labeling, 120
  in breast lesions, 116–117, 118f
  in bronchogenic carcinoma, 115
  contrast agents for, 113
  in kidney disorders, 121
  in liver lesions, 117, 119f–120f, 120
  in musculoskeletal tumors, 122, 124f
  in myocardial infarction, 115–116, 116f
  in pelvic carcinomas, 122, 123f